Reconceiving Women

Reconceiving Women
Separating Motherhood from Female Identity

MARDY S. IRELAND

THE GUILFORD PRESS
New York   London

Library of Congress Cataloging-in-Publication Data

Ireland, Mardy S.
　　Reconceiving women: separating motherhood from female identity /
Mardy S. Ireland
　　　　p.　cm.
　　Includes bibliographical references and index.
　　ISBN 0-89862-123-2　　—　　ISBN 0-89862-016-3 (pbk.)
　　1. Childlessness—Social aspects—United States.
　　2. Childlessness—Psychological aspects.　3. Women—Psychology.
　　4. Birth control—United States.　I. Title.
HQ755.8.I64　1993
305.48'904—dc20
　　　　　　　　　　　　　　　　　　　　　　　　92-45776
　　　　　　　　　　　　　　　　　　　　　　　　CIP

*For my parents
and David W.*

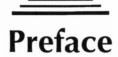

Preface

The Pacific Ocean separated their everyday lives, but on this day the two friends were engaged in a prolonged conversation. Having browsed through a bookstore prior to meeting for lunch, the visiting friend expressed her disappointment in picking up a book concerning women in midlife and not finding a single chapter which reflected her concerns, her feelings, her life. "It's as if everyone is a mother! Where are the books about us? What about our lives?"

My visiting friend was a 46-year-old professor of early childhood education. I was a 39-year-old psychologist. Both of us were in what many would call maternal occupations, though neither of us was a mother. For my friend, the timing of career, relationship, and motherhood never meshed; for me, delay and infertility were the reasons.

That day at lunch I realized for the first time that childlessness can be about many things. It is about biological limitations. It is about ambivalence. Sometimes childlessness is just about wanting something else in life. And sometimes childlessness is a combination of all these things.

The reasons for living a life without parenthood are personal and individual, but the term "childless woman" seems to be based on societal and gender role expectations. Where do I, my friend, and all other childless women fit in society? Do we have a place? We began to wonder about definitions of womanhood that result in the view that women cannot be complete without children, and how the growing number of childless women in today's world define themselves and establish their identities.

The search for actual women to interview became an individual effort of networking among colleagues and friends in the San Francisco Bay Area. When my university issued a brief press release regarding my research project, then titled "Invisible Women," it became apparent that the question of the meaning and place of women who are not mothers resonated with large numbers of women. A news anchorwoman's personal interest in women choosing not to become mothers resulted in a television interview. Following this local media exposure, I was deluged with telephone calls; more women than I could possibly interview responded. This book is the result of talking with 105 of the women who expressed interest in being part of this project.

During the course of the interviews, analysis, and writing of this book, the project titled changed from "Invisible Women." It became clear that only some women without children felt "invisible" in society. Some women felt all too visible. Yet all of the women, in varying degrees and in varying circumstances, perceived that others experienced them as a source of discomfort because their lives lay outside the parameters of traditional womanhood. Thus "Reconceiving Women: Separating Motherhood from Female Identity" became the title of this book about and for them, in an effort to add more words to the meaning of women's many different lives.

Acknowledgments

Over the course of the five years it has taken to complete this project, many people have accompanied me and given their assistance. My foremost and deepest appreciation extends to all the women who responded to my request for interviews, and were willing to take me into their homes and offices and talk to me at length about their lives.

My special thanks to Anna Chavez, whose personal and professional interest in this topic provided me with a public forum that facilitated contact with many of the women I interviewed.

A number of friends and colleagues made themselves available to discuss ideas on long walks and/or to read portions of the manuscript during its evolution: Beverly Burch, Lynn Franco, Matt Weissman, Amy Weston, Kathy Mill, Jean Dixen, Chuck Brandes, Sue Elkind, Kate Parker, and Sara Hartley. My heartfelt appreciation for their input and support.

Sandi Tatman's intuitive compatibility and editing skills helped shape my ideas and my writing—I could not have done it without her.

Kitty Moore, my editor, saw into the thicket of this work and helped me untangle its knots. She made the writing process an enjoyable one to be engaged in.

The work and teaching of analysts Andre Patsalides and Tom Ogden have been a persistent presence in my thinking.

My writer's group (Karen Johnson, Teresa Lebeiko, Diana Morgan) lovingly provided the perfect "holding environment" through all the stages of this project.

Lillian Rubin's work inspired this research. Her mentoring and friendship throughout the project added immeasurably to its completion.

Without Stephanie Feeney's enthusiasm for our idea, her consistent emotional support when other work drew her energy elsewhere, and her steadfast belief in the importance of my completing the book, it would have never been finished.

Finally, two people generously gave essential emotional and material support in ways that made it possible for me to begin and complete this project. Brad Gascoigne, who recognized the meaning of this work for my life, was seminal in his contribution at the beginning and middle stages. Suzanne Miller, with her lioness heart and hearth, guaranteed its conclusion.

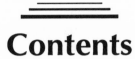

Contents

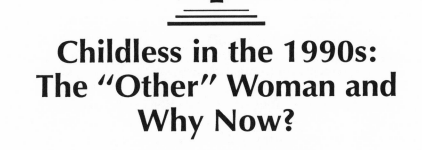

Childless in the 1990s:
The "Other" Woman and
Why Now?

Women have got to have a sense that there is something they
can bring forth, but how that happens is a question. . . . The
experience of bringing something forth is what is critical, but
there are different pathways to it.

    The path of the mother is easier in that there is more
known to it even though you have to be receptive and open to
the uniqueness of that particular child, while the non-mother
has to find her way more obliquely by trial and error and by
guidance from her unconscious.
                  —A 40-year-old woman childless by choice

It is nearly impossible to think about the adult woman who is not a
mother without the spectre of "absence." Why? Having a child
makes a girl a mother—it doesn't necessarily make her an adult
woman. Yet there is an implicit assumption that motherhood is
intrinsic to adult female identity. This assumption necessarily
implies an "absence" for any woman who is then not a mother.

    Rather than viewing the woman who is not a mother as missing
something, let us look instead for what is absent from our usual
conceptions of womanhood. Only when the assumption that all
girls must become mothers to fulfill female adulthood is challenged
will a woman's destiny truly be her own.

    It is impossible to get an accurate figure regarding the total number of American women who are not mothers because statistics regarding women's childlessness are compiled only on women of childbearing age. Some recent figures help. In 1988, 38% of American women between the ages of 18 and 44 were childless. In the 30–34 age group, 25% were childless, and in the 35 to 39 age group, 18% were childless. This is a 150% higher rate of childlessness than reported by women of these same ages in a similar survey in 1976.[1]

A small body of literature about women who are not mothers has been slowly evolving over the last 20 years (see Appendix), but there has been surprisingly little recognition of their social presence and psychic reality.[2] These women have been virtually omitted from everyday conversation and media accounts of women's lives.[3] (Despite the full life of Murphy Brown, the news anchorwoman of the popular television show by the same name, it was apparently deemed necessary to make her a mother in 1992.) There remains considerable ambiguity about why a woman becomes and remains childless. A number of historical and social changes seem to have contributed to the increase in childlessness.

Female Identity in a Changing Sociological Context

Prior to the 20th century the primary assumption in America regarding women's childlessness was that it must be due to infertility or poor health.[4] Voluntary childlessness among women really became possible only in the early part of this century, with the changes brought about by urban industrialization. This urban shift created more jobs for women. Along with the first birth control clinics and the suffragette movement promoting women's rights, a changing cultural context resulted in women without children emerging as a social and psychological phenomenon.

During World War II a generation of American women was intensely encouraged to work, and then just as stongly courted to resume homemaking, as returning servicemen reclaimed "their place" in the work world. Family size increased during the postwar decade of the 1950s, although prior to this decade fertility had been on a general decline. This change in birthrate can be at least partially attributed to the concerted efforts of Madison Avenue's advertising campaign to return women to their rightful place as mothers.

The "baby-boom" daughters of this generation of women carried into young adulthood their mother's unconscious (and sometimes conscious) wishes for something besides motherhood.[5] Given the backdrop of women's experiences from World War II, it is perhaps not surprising that a second wave of feminism broke upon the shores of public consciousness in the 1960s, producing a significant number of women who did not become mothers. Unlike the first wave of feminists in the 1920s, who had sought rights for women through championing motherhood, women in this second wave instead demanded rights more through promoting the alternatives to motherhood.

The 1960s witnessed dramatic changes in views on race, sexuality, the meaning of war, gender roles, and so forth. For the children of the postwar, baby-boom generation, the 1960s were the time of "the origin of the myth of that tribe"—a myth that one could strive to be individually authentic, yet remain a connected and contributing member of one's community.[6]

In this period the usual notions of coming of age were altered. All previous forms of established thought and behavior were challenged. It could be said that this decade captured the spirit of our postmodern era, in that postmodernist thought and discourse strive "to make us skeptical about the ideas concerning truth, knowledge, power, history, self, and language that are often taken for granted within and serve as legitimations for contemporary Western culture."[7] "The premise of the 1960s was that everything was possible and therefore it was important to think, because ideas have consequences."[8] What had been taken for granted by the previous generation was no longer necessarily so. This feeling, however naive it may appear now, was reflected in the words of a 43-year-old woman I interviewed who had been active in civil rights and other political movements, had served in the Peace Corps, and had later lived in a communal house with her husband:

The world was ours to make. . . . It was an enormous mantle, the responsibility to live as we believed. You don't just articulate ideas, you follow through with them. You think about what you want and then you really go and live it.

Many women were involved in one or more political movements during those tumultuous times. "I was really involved in the
Chicano movement, the farm workers movements, the antiwar
movement. . . . I was just very active," proclaimed a 39-year-old
woman I spoke with. She had organized Chicana women on her
college campus to respond to the cafeteria's unwillingness to buy
union lettuce. The women cooked and sold alternative lunches on
campus, "with not a lot of support from Chicano men," she added
with a grin. (It was, I might add, a successful effort.)

The ideas and values of the beginning women's movement
affected not only many women's youth, but became integral to their
older adult identities. Two-thirds of the women whose lives are the
basis for this book said that they were in some way involved in the
activities of those times, and one-third of them mentioned either the
1960s, or a significant feature of it, as "one of the most influential
factors" in shaping their adult identities. Many believed that their
identities were somehow anchored in the events of this time period.
One 39-year-old woman summarized these feelings:

> It was my good luck to have been born in a certain time in the
> culture, [one] where my natural inclinations were accepted.
> Over time, there became a place for me. It may not have been
> there in 1948 when I was born or in the fifties when I was
> growing up, but by the sixties there was a place for me. . . . If I
> had been born earlier . . . I'm sure I would have children and I'm
> sure I wouldn't have been a doctor.

The woman who had organized Chicana women on her campus
summed it up concisely: "My whole constitution was formed by
those times."

Thus the radically shifting cultural landscape of the second half
of the 20th century permitted these daughters to sidestep the
limited female identity their mothers were less able to overcome:
the view of the female as the desired object who waits—waits for a
man to choose her, thereby giving her status and definition as a
"Mrs." in relation her man. These daughters were instead able to
step into an unknown space and begin to define female identity in
new, different, and personal terms. For example, "Black is
beautiful," "gay," "Ms.," and the retention of their maiden names

by married women were all attempts to reconstruct social perceptions through changes in language.

Abortion rights were (and are) central to new personal freedoms for women and the emergence of different female identities. Before effective birth control, to be a woman and be sexual was to become a mother, but to become a mother was to become nonsexual. The young women of the 1960s and early 1970s challenged this collective paradox and highlighted the difference between a woman's reproductive capacity and her sexuality; the meaning of this difference is still evolving.[9] Heterosexual women who are mothers and are pro-choice in part emphasize the difference between female sexual desire and a maternal desire. The increase of lesbian mothers also denotes the psychic separation between female sexuality and maternity. Yet another element of this continuing sexual evolution is represented in the lives of women who are not mothers, whose sexual desire cannot be easily eclipsed or ignored by society because attention cannot be focused on their mothering functions.

The significance of abortion rights for women is emphasized by the fact that approximately 50% of the women interviewed for this book would probably be mothers now if these rights did not exist; 50% of them had had abortions. Although not all women who had abortions consciously intended to remain childless, virtually *none* of these women, in hindsight, would have altered their decisions. Negative emotional consequences of abortion among these women were associated with illegal abortions occurring prior to 1973. This finding was particularly important in the 1980s, when women faced a serious threat to their personal freedom and pathways to female identity because of legislative and judicial sanctions limiting legalized abortions. These threats are being reduced by the Clinton administration. Recent studies have shown that many women denied abortion have negative feelings that may last for years, whereas the children born when the abortion is denied have "broad based difficulties in social, interpersonal, and occupational functions."[10] It has never been so clear that recent judicial and legislative events foreshadow a contemporary political and emotional referendum on whether woman's (and man's) identity will remain tied to the concept of motherhood as woman's "manifest destiny."[11]

Effective birth control and abortion rights have meant delayed childbearing, which has produced a generation of older mothers who are bringing new and interesting dimensions to women and midlife, resulting in changes in the way we speak about motherhood. But delaying childbirth has also meant that some women do not have children at all. Despite the fact that in 1988 women between the ages of 40 and 44 represented 16% of all women of childbearing age, they accounted for only 2% of all births that year.[12] Although delayed childbearing has become more common, and perhaps even fashionable, some women expecting to have a child in their late 30s or even 40s will simply not be able to, because of infertility problems or other limiting circumstances. For another group of women, waiting results in unintended childlessness, when they find themselves at the end of their childbearing years without a child. For yet another group of women, delay has meant an ultimate decision not to have a child at all. These are all women who are not mothers.

One way of viewing the current circumstances of these women's lives is as a "third wave" of feminism; one in which motherhood is only one important facet of female identity, not necessarily central to development of woman's sense of her adult self.[13] Both the feminism of the early 20th century and the second wave of feminism in the 1960s were influenced by the idea of motherhood as central for defining female identity, albeit in different ways. The suffragette movement embraced it as a means to broaden and expand women's rights. The women's movement in the 1960s reacted to the centrality of motherhood by championing all other alternatives. The 1970s then gave rise to the concept of androgyny, based on a definition of human characteristics as particular to one sex or another, with the androgynous individual exhibiting characteristics of both sex roles. Now, in the 1990s, some intently question whether human characteristics need to be dichotomized and defined by gender at all. For women who are not mothers, paths of identity development increase when women do not have to be identified as opposite of men, but as both similar and truly different.

Female Identity in Psychological Theory

In myth and folklore we find a variety of contradictory descriptions of women who aren't mothers, but few are positive. Women who are not mothers are frequently described as women to be pitied (barren or unmarriagable) or as exceptional women. (Artemis or Athena in myth and real-life figures such as Anna Freud or Georgia O'Keeffe come to mind.) Alternatively women who are not mothers have been viewed negatively as selfish and unwilling to fulfill their womanly natural function. In this regard witches throughout history represent this version of the feminine, as women to be feared—powerful, self-serving, usually child-hating, and a threat to the institutions of society. How do we understand these rather extreme interpretations of this "other woman?"

Classical psychoanalytic theory regarding female development has justified and supported a portrayal of women who aren't mothers as deficient or negative, viewing them as unable or unwilling to fulfill a feminine role. Since psychoanalysis is the most significant psychological perspective in this century, shaping our understanding of the human psyche, the impact of this negative and incomplete portrayal of female identity has been substantial. (See Chapter 5 for a summary of psychoanalytic and other psychological perspectives on female development.) Male reproductive functioning and fatherhood are not the centerpieces for adult male developmental theory, but female reproductive capacity has become central and definitive for normative female development. Maternity has been the cornerstone of the mature adult identity for women. However, as childlessness becomes an increasingly visible option for women, the question of female identity apart from motherhood becomes increasingly difficult to disregard or patholo-gize. The woman who does not have motherhood as a positive adult female identity has been, and is, a complication in our theories of female development.

At the end of the 19th century less than 10% of women were childless; this figure is closer to 20% near the end of this century, and some researchers predict it will be higher.[14] No woman, mother or not, will ever be free to fully explore her capacities as a human being if the only valid role in which to feel she is an adult or a "real woman" is that of a mother. A woman should not have to be left feeling that she has a hole in her identity, is unnatural, or is threatening to others simply because she is not a mother.

A broader view of female development that could incorporate aspects of nurturance and personal empowerment would result in a conceptualization of women as different equals of men. The presence of a larger group of women who are not mothers evinces a pressing need for this redefinition. The integration of female personal authority, sexuality, and multiplicity of desire into the concept of female identity would, however, inevitably result in a revising (and possibly a reintegration) of the gender-role dichotomies upon which much of our current social structure is still dependent.

Childless Women, Relationships, and Work: Common Myths

In Chapters 2–4 specific women's lives are explored to illustrate three different pathways to a different female identity. But before moving on there are two common cultural myths about "childless" women which need to be addressed: (1) Childless women do not value or are not as capable of sustaining personal relationships; (2) Childless women are overinvested in career or work.

Fictional characters such as Alex Forrester, the antagonist in *Fatal Attraction*, represent the most negative version and feared outcome of a stereotype of the childless woman: a socially isolated, career-driven woman consumed by a fatal jealousy and envy of motherhood and the nuclear family. Portrayals such as these imply a subtle (and occasionally obvious) belief that women who are not mothers must have fewer and/or poorer relationships, or at least value relationships less. Contrary to this belief, relatedness to others among the women I interviewed was both prominent and meaningful.

The vast majority of the women whose lives are the basis for this book mentioned relationships as one of the most formative influences of the past 25 years for their adult identities.[15] Relationships with lovers and friends contribute significantly to the creation and sustaining of an atypical (childless) female adult identity. Relationships can also help a woman confront the limitations of current ways of thinking about herself. In short, relationships are both the mortar which helps hold an identity together, and at times a catalyst for change.

The relationships described by the one hundred women I spoke to reflect certain differences we have come to expect regarding female versus male attachments.[16] Women generally will say that relationships are very important, and place a great deal of emphasis on maintaining these connections; men often value relationships less and do less to maintain these connections. In particular, friendships for most women are an important source of intimacy or comfort; men have relationships centered more around their activities, like work or sports interests. There is also more personal attention given by women to their female friends than by men to their male buddies. Childlessness, it seems, does not make a significant difference in what appears to be a gender pattern of relating. In general the relationships of women who aren't mothers reflect our transitional times—times in which the boundaries defining and separating the gender roles of women and men have become more flexible—and times in which the relationships between women themselves have become more differentiated.

Primary relationships are usually a vehicle of adult development for most women. Despite some differences in the primary or committed relationship patterns among the women interviewed here (discussed in detail in Chapters 2–4), depending whether their childlessness was by choice, delay, or infertility, the centrality of relationship for adult female identity remains a common theme. In particular, primary relationships among women who aren't mothers underscore a boundary between motherhood and female sexuality that is often either ignored altogether or overstated. This boundary confusion results in women's inheritance of two opposing models of female sexuality: the nonsexual mother or the sexual nymphomaniac. The primary relationships of these women do not support either of these constructions.

Women who are not mothers show clearly that love, female sexuality, and motherhood are not the same. Heterosexual women who love and sexually desire men and yet do not have a strong wish to become mothers engage in relationships that reveal a variety of forms. In addition, some homosexual women love and sexually desire other women yet also have the wish to become mothers. Both heterosexual and homosexual primary relationships of women illustrate that the salience of gender and gender role to a committed relationship depends greatly on the particular circumstances and couple involved, and is in no way constant across all relationships. The various roles taken by these couples within the relationship show that gender as an organizing concept may be more pertinent for couples with children than it is for two adults building a life together. In Chapter 7 I will explore the limitations and possibilities of a gendered view of identity.

Friendship

Approximately 61% of the women said that friendship had a very significant impact on their lives.[17] This impact can be formative as well as validating. For women who are not mothers, a network of women friends can be especially helpful in establishing and maintaining a positive sense of female identity in a society which provides minimal positive reflection of their identity and lifestyles. Just as the woman who consciously decides to have a child may do so in part as a result of seeing her friends bear children, another woman may see most of her friends remaining childless. Alternatively, a woman may *un*consciously seek out other women who are not mothers to support one side of her maternal ambivalence as a way of resolving her own questions regarding childbearing.

The role of friendship for consolidating identity is evident in the history of many of the women I interviewed. One 42-year-old woman was chronically ambivalent about motherhood. Like half of the women childless by delay, she had become pregnant once, but chose to have an abortion. Later, in her mid-30s, she tried insemination, which failed. She again changed her mind about having a child. Only after turning 40, which seemed to be her own self-imposed age limit, did the child issue seem, as she put it, "95% resolved." At this particular time she became aware of her increased desire and need for support for her lifestyle.

> Because all my friends have been struggling with the same issue, they have been very supportive and tend to want me to do whatever they've decided to do. I understand that, because when I see some friend of mine end up deciding not to have children, I feel validated in some way. And when someone does have a child I feel envy or longing, and "Oh, God, has this been a terrible mistake?" So I understand that wish to have other people come to the same conclusion. [What this woman has found over time is that] . . . none of my closest friends now have kids. And maybe some of this is that it's painful to be too closely

involved with them and their childrearing and family. And some of it is also that I don't want to, in a way that I don't like to, spend a lot of time with little children, and their little children are always there.

Clearly, friendships can shape identity. Friendship can also serve to mirror one's changing identity. Mirroring serves to reflect back to a woman the very identity she has worked hard to consolidate; it helps keep it stable.

As part of her conscious acceptance of her own childlessness, a woman will often seek to add to her life other childless women, or women who, though mothers, have a substantial investment in other social roles. Those women experiencing the most difficulty accepting their childless circumstances and coming to satisfactory terms with a personal identity from which motherhood is excluded are either those who are very isolated or those whose circle of friends includes only women who are mothers. The lack of any mirroring of their own childless lifestyle will almost invariably evoke feelings of incompleteness or deviance, or sometimes both.

The results of this lack of mirroring are poignantly expressed by a 46-year-old woman who, with her husband, had tried for years to overcome fertility problems through various medical interventions. At the time of the interview she was just beginning to accept her childless state. She had no childless friends in her support network. She said that recently she found herself reading the obituaries of childless women in the local newspaper, trying to find out what their lives had been like. Her curiosity was not due to a morbid fascination with death; it was a search for positive images of women who weren't mothers so she could begin to imagine a different life for herself.

For women who are not mothers, female friendship is crucial to the structuring of the very meaning of "woman," and provides a grounding of their atypical identities. Although the meaning of "woman" is provided in female friendship for women who are also mothers, friendship may not be as essential to them for grounding their female identities, because they have many historical definitions of woman as mother to which they can attach and ground their female identity. In conclusion, friendship is one vehicle of adult development in which, through a selective process of identification and complementarity, a woman expands the meaning and texture of her female adult life.

Work or Creative Labor

The other common myth about childless women is that they are overinvested in career or work. This myth can be reframed by considering that the overemphasis on women's capacity for maternal relationships has diminished social recognition of their capacities for developing other aspects of themselves. Freud is said to have defined the hallmarks of a healthy adult life as the capacity to love and to work, but this seems to be applied primarily to men. Traditional gender roles have prescribed that the focus of women's real work should be motherhood. The creative labor of the women interviewed here offers another way to look at the meaning of women in the work sphere. Women who are not mothers have their own creative spirits to birth and bring into the world. That these spirits are not in accordance with traditional views of women's creative experience is not necessarily a sign of their deviance, but rather an indication that traditional views are incomplete.

Clearly motherhood had inherently more meaning as the central adult identity for women when the infant mortality rate was high and when there were more obvious links between the biological capacities of men and women for survival.[18] (We see these two connections in relation to female identity even today among the poorer and nonindustrialized nations.) But as the infant mortality rate has decreased, and basic survival needs have become less and less tied to biological capacities, the underpinnings of motherhood as the only "real" female identity are revealed in the social and political context of patriarchy.

For some women, motherhood is not a personally meaningful expression of creativity; motherhood, however, has been idealized and institutionalized in our society as inextricably linked with women's creative capacity. Nonmaternal activities seemingly continue to be regarded in a "lesser" light. Many, if not most, women harbor these negative perceptions, if only unconsciously, and consequently suffer guilt for having impulses to love and work that are not satisfied by motherhood. For some mothers, and for all women who are not mothers, creative work takes a form other than maternity, and many struggle to reconcile their own sense of fulfillment with the historically prescribed modes of gratification. Maternal ambivalence is seen in some way as pathological, as a woman's denial of her "natural" impulses and inability to come to terms with her "real purpose"; hence our society provides but two alternatives to women—accept your "proper" gender role or turn away from it and adopt a masculine gender role. Motherhood and female personal identity are once again equated.

The women who spoke with me displayed several different creative work patterns. These patterns are in part related to how their childlessness is dealt with, and to the degree with which a woman has unconsciously viewed childbearing as the primary mode of personal creative self-expression. The woman childless by choice actively chooses to focus her creative energy in places other than motherhood; in doing so she makes an important contribution toward dissolving social confusion regarding woman's creative energy and her procreative capacity. The woman childless by delaying circumstances or by infertility starts from a different vantage point. For these women the process of becoming an adult woman who is not a mother involves a redistribution of their psychic energies—motherhood, however much it is included within a fantasy of an adult identity, must cease to be the focus of creative endeavor, and other roles that express their identities must be found or created. When there is not a redistribution of psychic energy, truly satisfactory resolutions of a "childless" reality will not occur and a blocking of one's creative energy, diminished social functioning, and a poorer sense of well-being results. A woman's inability to detach sufficiently from a identification of woman as mother can result in ongoing anguish and a chronic difficulty in investing in alternative roles.

Job or career is one focus of creative energy that has been relatively restricted for women until recent decades. Despite the greater opportunities now available to women, work is unfortunately still cast in second-best terms for female identity, and not viewed as a coequal option to motherhood. That it is becoming increasingly acceptable for women to find fulfillment in nonmaternal occupations does not seem to have substantially altered the underlying belief that these alternatives are substitutes for women's real purpose and source of personal fulfillment.

The myth that motherhood should be able to contain all of women's desires was exploded over 20 years ago by Betty Friedan in *The Feminine Mystique* and by the women's movement. Yet it remains difficult for women to evaluate the issue accurately when society continues to view motherhood as the most important endeavor for all women. What has been absent or missing in the inexorable equation of women and motherhood is the social recognition that women, like men, can develop healthy personal identities that do not include the role of parent.

"Other" Female Identities

Because the reference point for adult female identity has traditionally been motherhood, it is fair to say that all women begin their pathway to adult identity by positioning themselves toward motherhood—either positively or negatively. I use the words "position towards motherhood" here in terms of maternal desire— the individual human capacity to exercise choice in moving toward or away from a desired object, person, and so forth. The degree of maternal instinct, which implies a biological mandate, varies in intensity among women; it is not simply present or absent. Becoming a mother, traditionally seen as a direct expression of a biological instinct, is equally, if not more, related to an act of conscious or unconscious will to fulfill a maternal desire.

This brings us to the research which was the basis for this book. One hundred voluntarily and involuntarily childless women between the ages of 38 and 50 were given a written questionnaire and participated in an in-depth interview. On the basis of a questionnaire sent to the several hundred women who initially responded to my request for interviewees, three groups emerged: women who choose not to have children; women who delay the childbearing decision until too late; and those women who have health or infertility problems making pregnancy impossible. In interviews exploring the life experiences of these women, their positions relative to motherhood became an organizing principle, and a means of describing three separate, though at times overlapping, pathways to an adult identity. These three pathways will be presented as separate and distinct, though in reality they more truly represent interwoven threads of the fabric of a particular kind of female identity. Each represents a different perspective from which a woman responds to the social expectation of motherhood. However, each pathway exhibits certain characteristics or dynamics more prominently than the others. Many women would no doubt identify with more than one of these pathways.

The "traditional" woman (Chapter 2) has tried to fulfill the traditional maternal role but could not because of infertility or health problems:

> *It started with, "What have I done that is so wrong that I haven't been chosen to be a mother?" ... It has been a long time learning to live with this empty presence inside.*

The "transitional" woman (Chapter 3) became childless because of delay. These women delay making a decision[19] until it seems too late to have a child.

> *I always thought I would have children but somehow it just didn't happen. I didn't want to be a single parent, but the man I was with never seemed to be the "right" one.*

The "transformative" woman (Chapter 4) consciously chooses not to become a mother. These women actively decide not to have children,[20] but the decision may or may not be made later, in their 30s.

> *The major feeling was I don't necessarily want a child. In the beginning I kept looking to understand why I felt this way—what was the pathology? Hadn't I really been mothered enough? Don't I have enough love to give? Don't I have the capacity to handle the demands of needs of a child? What is it that's wrong?*

In our changing cultural context, which includes a significant number of women who are not mothers, social–psychological interpretations and corresponding myths of childlessness and female identity must change as well. This is a change that is only beginning to occur. The two important themes of relationship and creative labor, discussed here in terms of all the women interviewed, are primary strands used in unique ways by the specific "traditional," "transitional," and "transformative" women described in the next three chapters. These women used these areas to consolidate and construct their own atypical adult female identities—as women, but not mothers. It is to their individual pathways to adult identity that we now turn.

2

The Traditional Woman: Child**less**

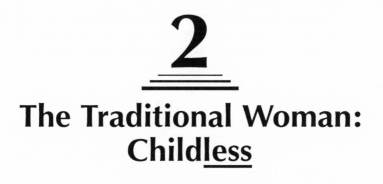

A woman at work lost a child and I almost feel jealous that she was lucky enough to have it nine months in the belly and six months as a living thing to love. I'm sorry as hell; I don't want them to lose it, but I think the loss of it without every having had it—it sounds so selfish—but it is a different kind of loss that is just as devastating. It's the loss of all the days together (with the child) and it's all the possible babies that you are also losing.

It could be that I haven't come to grips with [infertility] yet. Maybe once I can accept that, I can go ahead and be the "old me." . . . What I think I need is to allow myself to do some bona fide mourning. I just kind of hold that back, so I need to allow myself to do that. I think that this may be the "big thing" standing in my way to getting to my more open possibilities.

The "traditional" woman has said "yes" to motherhood, but her body has said "no." Most of these women experience themselves as child*less*, since motherhood has been prohibited by their poor health or infertility. Society is most familiar with and accepting of these child*less* women because they have desired but been biologically denied the adult identity of mother.

Each of the 100 women interviewed[1] completed the Bem Sex Role Inventory.[2] Traditional women endorsed a feminine sex role much more consistently than did women in either of the other two groups of childless women. A traditional feminine gender role identification is much more common among these women than among women from the other two pathways. This stronger identification with a stereotypical female gender role identity makes them more vulnerable to negative social judgments regarding their childless status. Some women interviewed said they felt like "defective women." It is as though this defect becomes painfully visible each time they reply "No, I don't" when asked whether they have children. Society's acceptance of and corresponding pity for these women may well reinforce their sense of being defective.

The central issue among these women is one of mourning. They must grieve the real loss of their physical integrity, the loss of their anticipated child, and the loss of their imagined identities as mothers. This mourning process is necessary if the traditional woman is to be able to view herself and others like her in positive, rather than damaged, terms. The mourning of any loss, physical or psychological, involves a process that moves from denial of the reality of the loss through acceptance of that reality to a new position of integration. In the case of childlessness, the new position that must be achieved is one in which a positive female identity and sense of self as complete can be maintained despite the exclusion of the possibility of motherhood from this self-concept.

The longer a woman pursues pregnancy unsuccessfully, the longer it may take for the mourning period to be resolved. It is as if each new fertility treatment, each attempt to conceive is a new experience of loss. One 47-year-old woman who at first felt she "wasn't a whole person" without children went through years of fertility treatment and surgeries. It was only after she stopped these efforts and began a true mourning process that she was eventually able "answer the question [about having children] without so much pain." In looking at this woman's experience we could say she was involved in an extended period of denial regarding her infertility, before shifting to acceptance that permitted her to begin to transform the pain of the loss.

Traditional women who seek to overcome infertility often confront the reality of motherhood as a political institution. Racism, heterosexism, and ageism can all come into play when a women who is unable to become pregnant seeks social assistance. The rate of infertility in women of color is one and a half times greater than in Caucasian women; yet only a small number of minority women actually seek infertility services, in part because of the prohibitive costs of these services.³ Women of color are also more frequently victims of hysterectomies than are Caucasian women. Two women in this study reported being sterilized without consent during routine surgical procedures for gynecological health problems; one of these cases resulted in a failed malpractice suit.

One woman I spoke with related that she and her husband had tried to conceive over a period of time, then attempted, in their late 30s, to adopt, only to be told that they were by this time too old to adopt an infant; they did not want to adopt an older child. Another 46-year-old woman told me she was denied infertility treatment when she was 34 because she was unmarried. Two years later, when she tried to donate her ova as one means of fulfilling some measure of her desire to procreate, she was again denied, this time because her "eggs were too old." Both women lived in the San Francisco Bay area, considered to be a very "liberal" part of the country. Conditions for adoption are less restrictive now.

Whether we agree with these social policies or not, each story suggests that traditional women can experience a double stigma that other childless women do not. Not only do they lack the social recognition accorded women who are mothers, but, when they seek to overcome their childlessness, they may be told that society believes they shouldn't have been mothers anyway!

Traditional women have tried to fulfill their female identities (at least in part) as mothers, and failed. Of all childless women, they may experience the most anguish. Unlike the "transitional" or "transformative" woman who, if needed to buoy their female identities, can maintain the fantasy that they "could have had a child," these traditional women cannot sustain such an illusion. Their empty womb may be perceived as a vast, unfillable, black hole. These women, in a very literal way, confront the task of unhooking reproductive capacity from female identity.

For the traditional women who had intended to follow a path to motherhood but could not, feminism has provided a cultural context in which they can begin to detach feminine identity from reproductive capacity and the institution of motherhood. For the first time, they don't have to feel *deficient*. A major impact of feminism for infertile women has been to help them realize that, in the words of one of them, "there is more to life than motherhood." Diane, the

45-year-old traditional woman described in this chapter, discovered her infertility at the age of 24, and initially expressed despair at not being "chosen" to have a child. Later she said of herself:

> I was really an ultra-conservative and worked for Goldwater. ... It was only later, in graduate school, that I really discovered myself, the woman–child inside, and feminism. And it was feminism that helped me to separate myself as a woman from my infertility.

For women whose discovery of infertility came later in life, feminism was a supportive foundation on which they could construct alternative ways of viewing and shaping their lives. One 42-year-old woman had required a hysterectomy at the age of 30 as a result of physical problems associated with the use of an IUD. Her husband was against adoption and was quite unsupportive; following her surgery he called her "half a woman." They divorced a year later. A subsequent relationship also ended when the man discovered she could not bear children. After two emotionally bruising encounters, she drew on the meaning and values of feminism to help restore her female identity. Since the women's movement championed alternatives to motherhood, she found it easier to affirm the pursuit of aspects of herself other than motherhood. She temporarily borrowed a "child-free" identity, telling others she didn't want children, rather than that she was unable to bear them. By the time she was 40, however, she was more able to speak about her childlessness in all its complexity.

> No one ever told me that having a hysterectomy didn't make me a woman. So after a while I got smart and just told men I didn't want any kids, because this seemed better. Now I am able to tell my story of the Dalkon Shield, my marriage, and my anger and disappointment about the whole thing, if anyone really wants to know.

Traditional Women and Primary Relationships

The primary relationship commitments of all the childless women interviewed emphasize the way in which their paths are different from those of their mothers. Of the 31 traditional women, 22 were currently married, three were living with a partner (one lesbian, two heterosexual), and six were single. Twelve had been previously divorced. Marriages among these women suffer when a child is hoped for but pregnancy or other means of having a child fail. One 39-year-old woman described the impact of infertility on her marriage:

> We both feel like eunuchs. I've felt like our relationship is really empty. . . . I feel like both my husband and I go around like these "lovesick cows" for children. We look at little kids and think how lucky [their parents] are. It's really hard. It is really hard for my husband because the realization is starting to hit him that it might not happen for us.

When raising children is presumed to be the major activity of a marriage, the realization that this will not take place shakes both the husband's and wife's gender and personal identities. (One woman said her husband was so upset over their inability to have children that, for a while, he lied to strangers, saying he did have children.) In our society, parenting is still attached more strongly to a *woman's* identity and gender role; regardless of whether or not she is infertile, the woman frequently bears the emotional stigma of a couple's infertility. For some of the women I interviewed, the primary relationship did not survive the crisis of infertility, because the burden could not be shouldered and worked through together. This was certainly a factor for Diane and her husband, whose story appears in this chapter.

When a woman finds herself to be infertile, she often cycles through a series of feelings and ideas about her infertility and its consequences for her identity. A mourning period is required in order that she may adequately reestablish her sense of self. The support of her mate is crucial. If it is not available, the process of arriving at a stable sense of self can be prolonged.

While the responses of family and friends to a woman's infertility are important, the response of a mate is critical for the reevaluation of the childless woman's identity. Her mate's response needs to validate her own wish to be seen as a whole woman, even without children. When this type of response is not forthcoming, coming to terms with a new sense of self is made more difficult.

Among the traditional women I interviewed, those relationships which weathered the crisis of infertility showed a capacity
for role flexibility. Both partners were able to shift from traditional
gender role expectations and try out new ways of being and doing
in the relationship. Men who can shift into roles that support their
wive's redirection of maternal wishes facilitate this needed transition. Women who can make the transition of shifting their creative
energy into roles other than motherhood can take advantage of this
flexibility. Their mutual capacity for change facilitates the needed
shift in the relationship's direction.

This kind of positive transition process occured with Martina
and her husband, discussed in this chapter. When flexibility is not
present, the relationship does not survive the infertility crisis very
well, if at all, and it will generally take a woman longer to reorient
her female identity into a satisfying, nonmaternal sense of self.

Traditional Women and Creative Labors

*I am someone who wanted to have children and a fairly
traditional woman's life, but things did not work out that way
for a variety of reasons and I have had to adjust my
expectations. I am one of a growing number of women who
face the spectre of infertility. We each have to work out our
own creative solution to this problem. . . . Mine has been to
abandon the dream of children and to opt for a professional life
geared toward care-giving and a personal life geared toward
learning.*

The traditional woman is one who invested a major part of her
self-definition in motherhood, but at some point found herself
incapable of bearing children. The traditional woman could be
termed the "reluctant career woman." Sixteen of the traditional
women in this study were professionals, eleven were nonprofessionals, two were students, and two were unemployed. More often
than in the other two groups, the women in this group began
adulthood with the idea that their primary role would be that of
mother; they thus assigned their work (if they worked) a secondary
status. Traditional women go through a process of reorientation
toward their work. When infertility or health problems prohibited

childbearing, these women often turned to developing a career as a second choice.

Diane, the 45-year-old traditional woman whose life is described in this chapter, felt that her work as a nurse had become a strong focal point for her creative energy and identity, but this was not what she had truly wanted for her life:

> *I never intended to have a career out of it. I never really had a desire for a career; all I really wanted to do was to be a mom. . . . Now my work is the biggest piece of my identity.*

Another 42-year-old traditional woman's infertility left her feeling a void in her life. Although she was already working, she found volunteer work with an organization devoted to world peace to be her choice for creative labor:

> *One of the major things that has helped me [deal with infertility] is that I have a way that I feel I can add positively to the next generation. It's not physical, like having children is a physical way you can add to the next generation. . . . But I've found a way to do that in another realm that isn't physical. And that is the most important reason why I feel really settled.*

Creative work addresses the sense of "something missing" that some infertile women (as well as some women childless by "delay") viscerally experience when they recognize their inability to fulfill their creative potential by being mothers. For this woman, meaningful volunteer work, helpful to the next generation to which she will not contribute a child, became an emotional, if not physical, experience of motherhood. This creative activity also fulfilled the need to nurture future generations by using one's knowledge and abilities to provide them with a more adequate social environment.

One-half of the traditional women reported having a mentor, while one-third of both the transformative and transitional women reported having a mentor relationship sometime during their work life. Mentors were people in these women's lives who extended themselves professionally, and sometimes personally, to encourage or directly support the advancement of their careers. One 40-year old woman I spoke with said she did not think she would become a professional when she married in her 20s. A hysterectomy necessitated by uterine cancer in her 30s put an end to plans to have a family. During these years she worked as a secretary. Mentoring from her boss enabled her to move up in the organization and eventually return to school to earn an MBA, leading to her current position in a marketing firm. As a women who came from a family that did not significantly value achievement, her own desires in the realm of work were significantly enhanced and supported by a mentor relationship with someone who could encourage her potential. The development of professional work did not substitute for motherhood per se, because creative energy can be focused in more than one direction, but in this situation her work absorbed and utilized the creative energy that could not be channeled toward motherhood.

Another 44-year-old woman said that mentors in her life had been instrumental in helping her develop work as a creative endeavor. Currently a technical writer, she had begun as a word processor.

> One mentor was my boss. She always encouraged me to "go for it" and I could ask her any questions I had on how I had to be or how I had to act to get where I needed to be, and she would tell me straightforward. And if it was something I just couldn't have, she would just tell me, "Don't bother, Mary, it won't happen." She could just know from the politics of the company or what was happening at the time.

Among the transformative and transitional women there is more individual interest and motivation to pursue nonmaternal work as a focus of creativity; hence they have less need for external validation of their choices. For the traditional women, however their primary choice of motherhood has been denied them, and nonmaternal work is a secondary choice; thus the traditional women reach out more often to others for support, mentoring, and validation, to facilitate their personal investment in creative labors other than mothering.

More than do the other childless women, the traditional women identify themselves with maternity; thus, for many of these women I found that their creative pursuits are more likely to have a substitutive quality, rather than being experienced as equally valid options. One 42-year-old woman who had had a hysterectomy at 29 and whose husband was not interested in adoption found that "being a super wife and supernurse" was going to "have to be OK" because she couldn't also be a "super mom." In expressing herself in this way she was placing an earlier identification ("always seeing myself as a mom and having kids") into a different nurturing *role* rather than shifting her identification to another focus. This is, of course, not true for all traditional women. Some of them are also ambivalent about motherhood and carry desires for other creative pursuits as well. For these women an infertility diagnosis can be used to resolve their maternal ambivalence in such a way as to unfetter the expression of their other creative energies.

Martina

Most of the interviews for this book were conducted in one of two places: in the women's homes or in their offices. I met with 38-year-old Martina in her home. As we sat at her dining room table I began the interview, as I did all the interviews, with an open-ended question: "Please begin with when the whole idea of being a mother or having children first came into your mind, and trace this until the present."

> One of the first things I can remember is that my mom was 15 when she had me. So one of the earliest things I remember my mom telling me is that she really wishes that I wouldn't get married and have children at a young age. She wished I would stay in school and do well. . . . So in my head, being a good girl, I said, "I'm going to do this."

Martina was the oldest of seven children in a Mexican-American working class family. As are many oldest daughters, she was a "second mom" to the other children, a role she still maintains with some of her siblings. She remembers the family as "stable," but "it also wasn't at times" because of her father's drinking. The effects of his drinking were mitigated by her mother's strong and reliable presence, her paternal grandparents (who also lived in the home), and by the large extended family that was always available. In retrospect, she saw her father as "doing his part by providing." Father lived and supported the values of justice and fairness, and he had the ability to acknowledge his mistakes. "He always said that all he wanted for his kids were to be people who know how to love people."

Martina's mother was and still is primarily identified as a mother to her children. Interestingly, a childless aunt was also an important member of Martina's extended family; "[someone who] coached us." She's the one people go to when they have their problems." This woman modeled for Martina a family role she now seems to have taken on for herself.

The issue of motherhood became a visceral reality when Martina became pregnant at 19. The pregnancy resulted from a relationship that she saw as having no future, so she decided to have an abortion. This was not an easy decision because of her Catholic upbringing, but "the whole concept of having a child seemed too risky to me." After seeing two doctors she was able to obtain a legal abortion, but found both the abortion and the efforts required to obtain it "a demeaning experience." The motherhood issue receded until, at 25 and while taking birth control pills, she unexpectedly again became pregnant. By this time abortion had been legalized and, because the relationship was a bicoastal one, she again decided to have an abortion. Although this abortion was easier to obtain, there was more guilt involved. I asked: "Did you wonder, what does this mean that it's happened again?" Did it raise some other questions about being a mother?" Martina picked up her glass of tea and began to swirl the ice uneasily as she answered:

> I thought about it, but not to a great extent. I was feeling a lot of things. I guess I just felt that I needed to be more responsible than the first time, but at twenty-five I didn't want to have a baby. . . . And, what was peculiar, right after that I became a Big Sister [in a Big Sister Program]. My little sister was a Native American young girl, We were beginning to develop this relationship. When I was twenty-five. This is weird. It was right after [the abortion]; I'm sure it had to be after. I'm kind of confused. But at twenty-five years old I became a foster parent, because this girl was having problems with her mother. That's what's kind of strange. I was terrified of being a mother to a baby, but yet I was totally willing to take on this kid. It was just an incredible experience.

In her confusion, Martina was realizing in this moment that there had been a connection between the abortion and her foster parenting—an unconscious atonement for the second pregnancy as well as a way of maintaining an identification with the maternal role. This foster parenting experience lasted a year; she later took on several more children over the next two years. Martina laughed as she said: "All this time my mom had said, 'don't get married young and have kids.' Only by the time I was twenty-eight or twenty-nine my mom was saying, 'come on, now, enough is enough.' "

When she was 28, Martina met her current husband through their mutual work in community social service agencies. They decided to delay childbearing for a while. Though they didn't use birth control, Martina did not become pregnant. After five years they decided to investigate the problem. A combination of events then occurred. Martina's husband was asked to complete a sperm test to see if the problem was his (because she had been pregnant before) and Martina was informed that previously diagnosed fibroid tumors had grown to such an extent that a hysterectomy was recommended. In shock, she immediately called her mother. Haltingly, and in tears, she described the conversation:

> So I said to her, "I guess you could say now I'm totally useless, because it's not like I have the sparkly shiny house for [my husband]. It's not like I do any of the traditionally womanly things. I mean, he does the cooking, and now I can't even do this." And my mother got real mad and said, "Don't ever think that. Having children isn't what makes you a woman." And this is a woman who had seven children. "Don't you see how much you give other people?"

Martina and her husband decided together that surgery was the best course of action. Their process of coming to terms with childlessness had begun. The adjustment has taken a period of several years. Two aspects of their relationship were advantageous: they shared a commitment to work and social values; and they also had a more egalitarian relationship than their parents, which gave them greater role flexibility. Martina mentioned that, one day, when her in-laws were talking about "a man's place," she piped in to say:

"Fortunately your son is strong enough to let me be strong, too, and he doesn't feel intimidated by that." Then there was total silence from them. If his feeling good depended on me feeling weak or less, that wouldn't be good. There are things that I'm a lot better and stronger at, and then there are things that he is better and stronger at. We give each other that. But it is not a matter of the fact that I'm a woman, that's why, or he is a man, that's why. We catch ourselves sometimes, however. It's true, certain things I just take for granted. It has to do with the fact that I've just been raised to expect [certain things from a man] and he does the same [about expecting certain things from a woman]. But when it comes down to it, there is some progress here.

Martina and her husband have had meaningful points of connection other than anticipating parenthood; they had the room to explore other ways of being in their relationship. This has been noticed by other friends:

One day my girlfriend said, "James doesn't know it, but he is actually a feminist, isn't he?" And he really is. It's been a struggle but, yeah, he doesn't just pay lip service. He really believes. I would feel comfortable if [we] had a daughter that he would be a good father to that daughter in that respect. He would react really strongly to any force out there that would tell her that she wasn't good enough because she was a girl or a woman.

Shortly after her surgery Martina quit her job in social service, a move which seems significant. She said that her quitting was due to the fact that she felt "burned out"; one wonders if she needed some unpressured time to adjust to the reality of her infertility. She took a job as a temporary, but very quickly this became a regular job in which she seemed to replicate her behavior following the second abortion. Of this new job, I asked: "So you, in other words, you adopted yourself a family?" and she replied: "Twenty-seven people, all ethnic backgrounds."

Martina again unconsciously compensated for her loss of fertility by finding another way to fulfill a caretaking role as she did when she became a foster parent after her second abortion. At another level we could interpret her move as taking an emotional "time out" from the creatively and emotionally demanding nature of social service work to absorb and digest her loss.

After two years of grieving Martina has moved into a position as a referral specialist. This, in part, satisfies her needs to be useful to others, and also satisfies her creative needs in a manner similar to previous positions. The work also allows her the flexibility of travelling with her husband (which is part of his job); this has added a great deal of satisfaction to both their lives.

At yet another level of her psyche Martina has come to terms with the reality of her infertility by altering her role in her family of origin. One of her sisters had volunteered to be a surrogate mother if Martina and her husband had so desired, but the couple decided against this option, and, Martina said:

Then I had this incredible urge toward my nieces and nephews. I thought to myself, "I have nephews and nieces and godchildren, and maybe that's what I'm supposed to be; maybe that's a good position for me to be in." And I was able to be satisfied with that. . . . Now I feel totally devoted to being with the kids and visiting the kids. . . . I enjoy the role of offering other things. . . . And I'm aware that I fill a place for the parents who can't always be present in the way the children need.

After a period of adjustment, her sisters have also come to realize this and appreciate that their children benefit in ways that would not have been possible were Martina to have had children of her own. In addition to her new relationship with children in her extended family, Martina creates a semiregular newsletter about and for the family; she and everyone else take great pleasure in this endeavor.

Martina's identity shift is also consolidating in the area of friendships. Until the last few years all her friends had children. She had been a part of a network of four families who did many things together over the years. Two summers ago, the families planned a camping trip. One of the group invited a number of additional people, assuming that Martina and her husband, having no children, would accommodate the newcomers at their campsite.

Her husband suggested that he and Martina stay at a nearby resort hotel and, instead, visit the campers. This was a pivotal experience for consolidating Martina's identity, as she said that "the reality is that we do live different lifestyles." Martina has since made an effort to expand her friendship network to include in her life women whose lifestyles are more similar to her own. That she has consolidated her identity as a child*less* woman is seen in her new response to colleagues:

> I don't know if it's just in my imagination, or just what I want to hear, but there's a lot of people I know who get pregnant. At my department alone there have been five or six pregnancies in a year and a half. What's happened is that they talk about having their babies and it is all wonderful. And then, afterwards, you hear nothing but complaints—"I don't get to sleep; I don't get to do this. She's biting everybody. She's doing that; she's doing this." I just kind of sit back and wonder. They say, "Are you sure you don't want to take my baby for a while?" And I know darn well that if anything happened to that baby, that they'd fall apart. I know that. But I also know that on a day-to-day level they get burnt out, and they get really frazzled. They see their own relationships deteriorate because of the child. The focus of their lives is just different after the birth than during pregnancy. I'm seeing two different women.

Upon hearing this, I asked: "Are you implying that part of what you get from these women is a certain amount of envy?" She replied:

> Yeah. It's one thing to say to so-and-so [who] doesn't have any children, "Oh, poor thing." But you can't say that if the person feels content and feels OK. Then it's, "What did you know that I didn't know?" comes out. . . . I really get a sense of how much sacrifice it is [to have children].

At this point in our interview I asked how she felt being a childless woman in today's society. Her reply indicated how important it can be to have a network for this atypical female identity, whether it is a supportive family (like hers) or other friends:

> Sometimes I get, "Why are you here if you aren't willing to bring someone else up the way you were brought up?" But the

way I think is: My mom had me; OK, that was her choice, her decision. And when she did, she didn't have me with the condition that I [would] turn around and do the same. She wanted me to be whatever I wanted to be. So I am not so influenced by society as much as I am by my own family and the freedom they give me.

At the end of our interview I asked Martina to imagine that she was a very old lady looking back at her life and evaluating it. How would she like to see her life? My purpose in asking this question was to understand the "big picture" perspective of each woman on her adult path, to determine if there were particular concerns about loneliness and regrets in old age. Martina's response seemed to address all of what I had, by implication, been asking:

I'd like to be able to feel that the younger people around me would feel that I was somebody who really lived. I may not have been someone who did great big important things, but lived and continued to have a pulse. . . . have some grace about me and still speak out. I don't feel I'll be lonely. My husband has some concerns about this. But if you are a warm, congenial person, and you're involved, you aren't going to be alone.

Martina has become a woman of her own, outside of the institution of motherhood, even though this is not what she had anticipated. She has mourned the loss of her potential identity as a mother. She shifted the creative, nurturing energy that would have been employed in motherhood into relationships with her nieces and nephews and into challenging and satisfying work and community service. In her own evolving process, the flexibility of her relationship with her husband was quite important. The support from her family as she moved into alternative roles was also a helpful factor. Finally, her move to develop female friendships with other nonmothers has enabled her not only to accept her childless circumstances but to view her atypical female identity as a valuable and meaningful one.

Martina's is only one pathway to identity for the traditional woman. Let us examine another woman's journey; one who is a few years older than Martina, and whose grieving process was more intense.

Diane

The walk to Diane's office was a long one, winding through hallways and across interior courtyards. When we reached her office, I was immediately struck by the calendar on her office door, filled with pictures of mothers and children. In what was otherwise a typical academic office, piled with papers and empty cups, atop her file cabinet stood a southwestern sculpture of a mother and infant.

> *I don't remember a time when I didn't want to be a mother. There's a picture of me at age three and a half which so succinctly captures my orientation and my raising that it's hard to believe. There's a picture of me with my tiny little ironing board ironing my doll's clothes. My doll is in the crib next to me, and there's a tea set. . . . I was raised to be a wife and mother. I never dreamed there was anything like an alternative lifestyle to being a mother.*
>
> *I think a diagnosis of infertility is, for many women, the kiss of death. At least I had career options. For very few woman are these much-touted drugs and infertility work-ups and stuff available. You basically have to be white middle class or a woman of color of upper class to get any of them. I wonder if little girls being raised now, whose moms are working, see that there are other options for them. I wonder what they feel. I wonder if they see themselves doing other things besides being mothers. I was really clear that I only went into nursing to pay for kid's teeth and the family room. I never really intended to have a career out of it.*

Diane was the adored only child of a lower-middle-class Anglo-American family. Her mother had tried to have other children, experiencing multiple miscarriages in her attempts to do so. As many of that generation, Diane's mother did not work, although she had harbored a wish to become a nurse. Diane's father managed a store. Both parents enjoyed parenting.

As her memory of the photograph indicates, Diane was very identified with her mother. As she saw it, "I was clear on my role from day one. I never would have dreamed of fixing a car, or my bike." Diane felt, in retrospect, that perhaps she was "too much the center of her mother's world." Though she believed herself to have been close to both parents, Diane felt perhaps a bit emotionally closer to her father. He had always wanted a daughter, and she shared many activities with him:

> *My dad and I used to go for walks every weekend. He introduced me to nature. He was always there to listen to me. He always wanted a girl; he didn't want boys. He was just wonderful with me. I thought the sun rose and set on him. . . . I remember him saying to me a lot of times, "Remember that you are no better and no worse than anybody else." When he died, it was the second biggest pain in my life, equal to my not being able to have children.*

Both parents stressed the primary values of education, hard work, and openness to diversity. These values were a mainstay for Diane in her later years, when she found herself upon a very different life course than the one she had anticipated. In addition to her parents and their values, she recalls two significant adults in her early life: her grandmother, and a woman friend of her parents. Both made her feel valued, and she looked upon both as female models. Of her mother's friend, she told me:

> *I realized a few years ago she was a lesbian. The word "gay" was never mentioned, although it was talked about that she lived with this woman and helped raise her kids. But I never got it. She was a nurse, and I thought she was wonderful. She used to come over in her nurse's uniform and they'd talk about hospitals and stuff. I thought that was just so neat. She, for a lot of reasons, probably helped me see that I wanted to be a nurse.*

Diane remembers being excited about beginning menstruation because then she "knew she could have babies." She also remembers being asked in eighth grade what she was most afraid of. One of her three answers was "not being able to have children." At 16 she began summer work as a ward clerk on the labor and delivery ward of a local hospital, before going to college. These memories clearly indicate that her desire for a family was present very early in her life.

After college Diane married a young man she had known since high school. When she was 24 they began to try to have a child. After six months with no success, Diane underwent a fertility work-up; the source of their infertility was discovered. It was initially believed that certain medications might be of help in this problem; over the next four years the couple continued to try to conceive. After these years of infertility treatments, a genetic abnormality in Diane's uterus was finally discovered; this brought the efforts to an end.

The stress of the infertility created problems in the marriage. Diane raised the issue of adoption, but her husband rejected this option. He did not want to raise someone else's child; he wanted his own.

I held myself in readiness to be pregnant for a lot of years. . . . I took only jobs, not careers. I was preparing myself to be a mother. I really truly expected I would be a mom. . . . Midway through that four years I took a teaching job, which was the first movement in my life that was the tiniest acknowledgement that "yes, I'm not going to be able to have children." . . . Prior to that I wasn't willing to take any job that I couldn't stop to have a baby.

Within a year of taking her teaching position, Diane's husband was transferred and the couple moved. In her new location she decided to return to graduate school for additional training in nursing. This shift in her life corresponded with the death of her father; this latter event propelled her into the world into a new way. Her father had always been, for her, "the real safety net." With his death she felt "I had to grow up," which meant developing for herself the qualities that she had previously looked to her father to provide. At this time the marriage began to unravel. The couple separated, with the husband moving to another area and Diane remaining in graduate school. This was the beginning of a gradual disengagement, though they remained legally married for some years to come.

Diane's years in graduate school were pivotal to her development as a woman who was not to be a mother. Her career began to shift from work that could easily be displaced for motherhood to a more substantive commitment. The school experience was also formative for her concept of self. Initially Diane viewed herself as "ultra-conservative and very Catholic." In graduate school she discovered feminism and, for the first time since her diagnosis of infertility, began to conceive of a personal identity beyond that of an infertile woman. Prior to this time Diane did not know any other infertile women; she was isolated and identified with a feeling of being damaged. Graduate school and feminism changed that:

> *I would have to credit those times and the people there with helping me put this infertility in some kind of perspective, because it truly consumed my whole life. [Graduate school] helped me see that I was separate from my infertility. [Previously] all I was was my infertility. It took over my whole world.*
>
> *At that point in graduate school I wrote twelve poems. In my second year of graduate school I sat down and wrote this poem [she showed me a poem about infertility] and I have never changed a word of it. Since then I haven't written a lot of poems, because that was evidently what I needed to write for.*

At that time all her closest friends had children. Since they were willing to share their children, Diane had the opportunity to, as she put it, "do some of the mom things." Since then she has also developed friendships with women who are not mothers.

After completing her degree, Diane and her husband reunited, and she obtained her first university appointment. When he was again transferred, she remained behind to continue teaching. Some months later, when her husband rejected marriage counseling, they agreed to a divorce. Within six months, he married a woman with a child.

Diane made a "political and intellectual decision" that she was a lesbian. She took a nursing position in another location, where she had her first sexual relationship with a woman. (A shift from a heterosexual orientation to a homosexual one is not an uncommon pathway for lesbian women.)

Diane's nursing career has been a significant part of how she has come to terms with the loss of her own childbearing capacity. She has involved herself deeply with the maternal experience in her pediatric work, teaching obstetrics and prenatal care. Her professional self is now a large part of her identity, but became so only in relationship to the growing realization that she would not be able to conceive or adopt a baby of her own.

Diane fought this realization at many levels. Even after her "coming out" as a lesbian, she did not give up her own desire to become a mother. Her female partner had no desire to bear a child, and the couple attempted to adopt a child. Their request for adoption was denied, not on the basis of their homosexuality, but because they had approached the adoption process as a "lesbian family":

> We were willing to take a disabled child. We went through the whole home study. They had us marked as a "couple." They didn't want us both to do it; they wanted only one of us to apply for adoption. It was an awful experience, just awful. I think, for me, when I finally realized [it wasn't going to happen] it brought all the stuff up again; you know, like one more time. Not only do you not get chosen by God or the universe, you don't get chosen by the county, either. So it was real hard.

This was to be Diane's "last gasp attempt" to get a child of her own.

> At that point I put it aside. I said, "That's it." There's no other opening, and I'm old. I mean, I'm forty-five now, and even though friends of ours have just adopted a baby and one of them is forty-five and the other is forty-seven . . . fine for them but not OK for me. The thought of being fifty and dragging a child into kindergarten was too much. Looking at being sixty-five and still working to put a kid through college was one thing, but being fifty and having a kid in kindergarten was more than I could handle.

Diane and her partner have recently provided a home for a 19-year-old lesbian. Tina, who had been living in a halfway house, was in need of financial support and guidance. Taking on this kind of maternal role has been a part of how Diane has accepted her childlessness. Diane reported that Tina is now enrolled in college and doing quite well. I asked how having Tina in her home has affected her.

[Not having children has] been a feeling of being an outsider. . . . One of the most wonderful things about having Tina live with us is that, on some level, I'm no longer totally excluded. For the very first time I saw the other side of having lost friends to babies because they no longer had time for their friends who didn't have kids. What I realize now is there is an incredible need to talk to experts. Not book experts, but people who are doing it. That has been a real gift, because for the very first time I get it, and don't take it so personally. While I still feel like an outsider in some ways, because of Tina I feel more like I belong. I feel awful about saying that because it is like trading on her, and I want to be totally altruistic about what having her in our life is like, and I'm not.

"But mothers aren't, either," I responded. "That's true, isn't it?" she replied, with an uncertain, shy smile of recognition.

At 45, Diane is beginning to accept and understand the effect of her infertility on her life, and her reactions to it:

Pain doesn't really explain it. It is a hollow, empty feeling of not being good enough, and it does a real number on your self-esteem. Of course, I did a real number on my self-esteem, or something about not being able to conceive. I think if I had been able to conceive and lose children, miscarry children, I think it would have been awful; but at least I wouldn't have felt like a failure as a woman. And I certainly did for a very long time. I don't any more. I think moving into a more feminist world, I think that really helped me put it into perspective. . . . Finally, finally, finally what happened, and the reason I can talk about it without sobbing, is that I finally made the choice. I chose. Because I could have gone on with a private adoption. But I finally made the choice that enough is enough, and I've done more than what is reasonable. I've done everything I can to be open to the universe, to be open to a soul coming into my body, to be open to (cries a little at this point). . . . It's just not going to happen. Around the time we got Tina I said, "That's it; I'm not willing to do any more." [This happened] when I was 45, so we're talking 21 years of carrying around the identity and the role, and the lack of presence inside me. It was really painful.

I'm really for the first time feeling congruent. Boy, it's taken a long time to get here. All the things I thought my life was going to about, like being married to an English teacher and having a lot of kids, being a grandma—that's not what my life is going to be about. And I've stopped fighting it. I've just said, "OK, this is what it is and it's really fine with me." I feel valued for what I do here [her work]. I am a gentle, giving person, and I'm on a spiritual path. I don't even know what to call that, except that it is not a religious experience, but very much connection with the cosmos, or whatever. And I feel like I'm able to give and share, and as long as I do that I will feel OK.

In developing a life different from the one she had expected to live, Diane has found points of feminine identification in her own mother's unfulfilled aspirations of becoming a nurse, as well as with her mother's close female friend who had been a nurse, and was also a lesbian. The points of identification alternative to motherhood were discovered in her significant friendships with women in her life, and with her current lover. She has reluctantly faced what had been lost to her, and has, over an extended period of time, created an alternative lifestyle that she, as a child, "had never dreamed of." Diane's life is filled with challenging, creative labor, and expression of maternal feelings, and a satisfying relationship. Her support of a needy young adult provides partial maternal satisfaction. Diane's life is very different from the one she expected to have, but it is a fulfilling one, forged from deep personal loss.

Conclusion

In selecting these two examples from minority women (racial and sexual) there was a risk that these women would be seen as somehow too atypical for traditional women. Non-Caucasian subcultures often place great emphasis on childbearing as a woman's pathway to identity; Martina's family supported her in her search for a nonmaternal identity. Lesbian women experience less social pressure to have children; Diane's pathway to accepting childlessness was a difficult and long journey. In a profound sense, however, both their lives, represent common experiences of women dealing with their maternal desires within the context of infertility.

The lives of these two women illustrate that a primary dynamic (but certainly not the only one) among traditional women is mourning, grieving, and accepting the loss of potential motherhood. For traditional women, being child*less* is a loss of varying intensity and poignancy. The working through of this loss is a circling arc of lessening emotional intensity spiraling through their lives, never entirely fading, as it provides some structuring function for development of adult identity.[4] The woman who can confront the loss of potential motherhood can use the lost potential as a well from which alternative creative endeavors will spring. In writing about the process of mourning, Freud noted that the ego could give up the lost/dead person only when significant features of this person were incorporated in some way into the grieving person's identity.[5]

The woman who discovers she is infertile does not become child*less* overnight. She must undergo a similar process, becoming child*less* over a period of time as she experiences moments of internal structural change. In these catalyzing moments, something inside her shifts to re-form her adult female identity without motherhood as part of its meaning. As her life unfolds it must appear not as a mere substitute for motherhood, but as a viable alternative pathway. She must broaden her identification with the feminine to include some aspects of woman not necessarily attached to maternity or family relationships. As she does this, her life will take on a different character, as we have seen in the lives of Martina and Diane.

Sometimes work or career will take on a different quality of importance and meaning. A woman's identity may shift as she withdraws energy previously invested in the concept of motherhood and places it elsewhere. When Martina changed jobs she took a position that involved her less in caretaking and more in creative leadership. Her flexible work schedule permitted her to include other meaningful things in her life, allowing her and her husband to experience their nonparental relationship in new ways.

Alternatively, a woman's identification with motherhood may not shift to other areas, but will be expressed in roles alternative to motherhood, retaining some measure the fulfillment of maternal identification. Such was the case with Diane who, upon accepting her ultimately child*less* situation, took on a foster parent role.

The traditional woman needs either to shift her identification away from the maternal, or to adjust her maternal identification by restructuring her social roles. This shift is facilitated by the support of family, friends, and significant others, most particularly the last. By accomplishing this shift she will be able to relinquish the fantasy of motherhood, give a form to her grief, and ultimately harness her available psychic energy to transform and redirect her life.

When a woman is unable to accomplish this shift, for whatever reasons, she will remain in a state of what could be called "pathological grief." Her experience of loss will continue unabated and will not be transformed. Under these circumstances she will continue to feel her feminine self is damaged and that her life is somehow less. She will be unable to identify herself as a woman who is not a mother but still a woman, with a full, satisfying life.

3

The Transitional Woman: Child-free and Childless

> I never thought of having children outside the context of a husband and home, and I just never met the "right" person to make it happen.

The women of the "transitional" pathway are living in the stream of social change. They want to pursue the social and career possibilities that are now open to women, but they also want, or think they might want, to have a family. Unlike the "traditional" women, this group identifies with characteristics of both feminine and masculine sex roles.[1] These women could be called androgynous, but in another sense they can be said to express an alternate female identity, rather than aspects of a male identity (which is implied by the term "androgyny").

For a number of reasons, "transitional" women delay childbearing until it is seemingly too late to have a child. Some women are trying to complete their education or establish their professional careers before having a family. Others have certain criteria in mind (financial stability or a particular vision of a committed relationship) that they are seeking to satisfy before motherhood, and that never come about. Still others are simply living their lives as they unfold, with the idea in mind that "some day" they may have a child. At some point, all are awakened by an internal voice or external event that calls their attention to the time line of their lives; they realize that motherhood is not going to happen.

41

Paradoxically, in the lives of transitional women the saliency of gender is highlighted and put within a context in which gender can be challenged as the most important category for structuring human experience. Parenthood influences the structure of women's lives far more than men's. Women are generally the primary caretakers of children. Choosing to be a parent affects a women's course of development far more than it does a man's, but whereas motherhood structures a good portion of a woman's life, it does not structure it entirely. In addition, the transitional woman's indecision or inability to create the "right" conditions for childbearing shapes a good portion of her life, but not its entirety.

To a greater or lesser extent, these women are ambivalent about the demands of motherhood. Some have difficulty acknowledging this ambivalence to themselves, which contributes to the delay. Others find themselves near the end of their childbearing years without a mate with whom to bear or raise a child, and feel that their childlessness is due to chance (see the quotation which begins this chapter).[2] Whether it is due to their own ambivalence, poor timing of relationships, or other formidable circumstances, at the close of their childbearing years all transitional women are faced with assessing their lives and, possibly, reorienting them.

Women who avoid addressing the delay into childlessness appear to have the most difficulty maintaining a positive and coherent sense of female identity. They often feel as though they are not fulfilling their own or society's expectations of what a woman "should" do. This blanket denial of the delay may take the form of a sustained illusion that motherhood will "somehow" be possible, an illusion that reproductive technology and the media are willing to support. Yet in these circumstances, without taking definite action to obtain a child, a woman drifts, getting older and older, never at the helm of her own life, losing opportunities to realize her creative and nurturing potential in other areas. In this respect transitional women can avoid the confrontation with their own childless circumstances in a way that infertile women cannot. Motherhood can appear to be included as one of her evolving, or serial, identities. The question is: At what point does the identity of mother become truly eclipsed?

Most women who become mothers do so before midlife. The childless woman who consciously evaluates herself in midlife has the opportunity to accept that her life seems to express some different desires from that of the woman who is a mother. Alternatively, she may experience her lack of being a mother as an unfulfilled desire, and will begin to address what it is that is "missing," interpret its meaning, and take some action to "fill" that missing space. This exploration will be similar to that of the "traditional" woman faced with infertility. It will involve acknowledging the losses not only of her imaginary children, but of the possible "selves" that might have developed through her experience of becoming and being a mother—selves which are now lost to her.[3] Once these losses are acknowledged, another creative focus and/or other nurturing activities become possible; she will be more able to absorb and integrate the loss that is particularly her own, in her own unique manner.

In addition to thinking about transitional women in terms of whether or not something is missing, we can also think of these women as manifesting a psychic struggle in which we all, men and women alike, are engaged. The transitional women's struggle between desires associated with the "masculine" or "feminine" can be expressed without recourse to gender by seeing each desire as a different subjective point of view regarding one's life experiences.[4] Any given moment of our experience can be understood in terms of the degree to which we are living in that immediate experience and the degree to which we are interpreting or defining that lived experience. Imagine walking by a bakery, seeing and smelling the baked goods. You can simply take in the pure experience of your senses, or you might begin to have memories, fantasies, and thoughts that begin to represent aspects of the meaning of this experience.

The "being in" experience has been traditionally identified with the feminine position, because of woman's perceived closeness to nature through her menstruation, pregnancy, and birth processes. The more abstract experience of putting language and interpretive understanding to human experience has been identified with the masculine position. Clearly, both women and men have both capacities; these two positions are not reflective of the physical body of femaleness or maleness but are inner subjective positions, both of which all human beings assume at different times in life.

The transitional women illustrate, in terms of motherhood, the shifting back and forth between these two subjective positions and their differing consequences for human lives. The shift between "going with the flow" of their lives and more active attempts to represent or interpret their desires for motherhood (and other pursuits) highlights the ongoing tension of trying to balance just living one's life and giving one's life particular meanings.

Because motherhood has been the central organizer of female identity, it is especially easy, in the lives of transitional women, to see the tensions and consequences for personal identity caused by shifting back and forth between these two subjective positions. For women, identifying with and unconsciously anticipating the socially expected role (motherhood) as an element in their lives is easier than addressing the meaning of the absence of motherhood or alternative "fullness." Generally it is only when her childbearing years appear to be at an end and/or there is no primary partner with whom to make a family possible that the transitional woman is required to address this question of meaning as an identity developmental task.

Women such as Karen and June, whose lives we will explore, live in a transitional space—somewhere between the past, when all women were expected to be solely or primarily mothers, and the future, where role and identity options for women will increasingly diversify into arenas previously reserved for men. Their processes in navigating this transitional space sharply detail the everyday struggle all of us contend with: the struggle between "being in" our lives (just living) and defining/interpreting our lives.

The cultural context of the 1960s and feminism provided the transitional women with an open field of possibilities to explore. For some, the loss of motherhood leaves an empty space in their lives, for others this space was filled by the possibilities provided by the changing times. Feminism bolstered a feeling that women's possibilities in life were endless; that women could somehow have it all—a life of their own and motherhood as well. Transitional women delay childbearing to explore themselves in a world which seems open to them. The pursuit of education, careers, relationships, and so forth are sometimes choices that represent much more of these women's identities than the part that desires motherhood. Realizing this fact in later life enables them to view their childlessness less as a loss and more as a recognition of a different sense of self. A 42-year-old transitional woman, born and raised in the south, said of her process in the 1960s and 1970s:

> *[My] twenties was a real struggle to grow up. I was doing all those things. I became very involved in political work. I became involved in the women's movement. I was part of a group that published a woman's journal. I worked in a free clinic. . . . I was connected with a rape crisis center. . . . I was active in community organizing sorts of things in the south. . . . I was involved in demonstrating against the Viet Nam war.*

Through her process of political and social activity, this woman began to separate her own identity from that of her family.

Another 42-year-old woman who was, at the time of the interview, trying to understand how her personal path as a childless woman had developed, typifies those transitional women who described themselves as "late bloomers." It is perhaps these women whose personal issues combined almost synergistically with the era in which they lived.

> *It was a very significant time for me. It was a coming of age that happened to dovetail with my marriage and a personal coming of age. I was involved in the antiwar movement, civil rights. . . . It just seemed that there was so much possibility and so much we could do.*
>
> *Then we left the country, which became more of a personal adventure and shifted away from the social. It was a very dynamic time. It was the most socially dynamic time in my lifetime.*
>
> *In the mid seventies when I was really going through whether this relationship [her marriage] was fulfilling or how we could make it so, of course the women's movement was so strong an awareness. I hate to look at . . . the decisions I made [in my life] as having been a result of some sort of social movement, but it was very much in sync.*

For some of these women who pursued all these new possibilities, there was a feeling that time was "forever young." They discovered only too painfully that time had eclipsed their capacity for motherhood. The deflation of feminism's heroic posture, the realization that women can't "have it all," fell perhaps most heavily upon these women. Yet feminism became a well from which they could draw when their delay into childlessness became an unexpected and rude reality. This is what one 46-year-old woman said of the two places and meanings of feminism for her life:

> The woman's movement meant a great deal to me. I was twenty-five or twenty-six years old and all of a sudden we were being told women can go out and have sex, too. . . . It helped me come out and do some of the things I always wanted to do and never felt that I could. I hadn't had the approval. The women's movement gave that to me. It gave me some validation . . . and told me I could just be as much as I could.

As for the residual impact on her:

> The woman's movement told women that they had to be independent. It told them that there are some things you are going to get in this life and some things you are not going to get in this life. And I think it's brought me to the place I am now. I'm OK where I am. . . . I have learned how to take care of myself, in every way—physically, emotionally, financially. I've learned how to take care of myself and the women's movement helped me do that.

Transitional Women and Primary Relationships

> It has just seemed that when I was with a man who might want children and be a good father I wasn't ready, and then when I was ready I seemed to be in a kind of relationship that was OK for me but not really one in which I would want to have a child.

It is in the relationship patterns of transitional women that we see most dramatically the interplay between family and society regarding gender roles. The "traditional" women desire more of a traditional relationship, and the women who choose a child-free life do not. The transitional women embody the conflicting desires of both groups. Among the 31 transitional women, only eight were married. Five were in committed relationships (three heterosexual and two lesbian) and 17 were single. Five women had previously been divorced. The pattern of serial monogamous relationships in this group is characterized by more brevity than the serial relationships in the other two groups; the transitional women stayed in relationships for a shorter period of time.

At one level these women's serial relationships (as do everyone's) reflect an attempt to resolve family relationship issues. In describing their adult development, these women used phrases like "late bloomer," or words with similar meaning. For many of these women, their inability to come to a final decision regarding motherhood or their inability to find a relationship they believed to be compatible with motherhood stemmed in part from the fact that their relationships reflected unresolved conflicts regarding their mother and/or father and their respective roles. These conflicts often express themselves in the selection of men who are not "father material," men who do not want children (or any more children), or men who have already had vasectomies. Each of these choices reveals a different level of maternal ambivalence and consciousness regarding the childless identity that follows from the choice. These women are, in effect, choosing to forego future maternal satisfaction for the present satisfaction of an intimate relationship, although this was often not acknowledged.

One 45-year-old woman avoided dealing with her own maternal ambivalence this way for a while, but later did return to truly process this as her own solution. Initially she believed that she had

> never really dealt with the issue of whether I will or I won't [have children]. It was just irrelevant. And when I met my husband at forty–forty-one he had had three children . . . and he had a vasectomy after his third child. The issue was then closed. I felt absolutely no grief or anything then about the fact that the issue was closed.

Later in our interview this same woman expressed a frequent sentiment of transitional women; that if she could redo anything about her childless circumstances she wished she had been able to sort out her maternal ambivalence sooner so as to have had more of a "real choice" about motherhood. In a similar fashion, June, the

woman we will meet later in this chapter essentially said that the
fact that she took longer in each of her developmental stages than
she would have like to had a significant bearing upon her remaining
childless.

It may be tempting to view the transitional woman's pattern of
relationship as being only a function of unresolved family issues
which interfere with her ability to establish a committed relationship. A corollary here is how rarely we are tempted to view
long-term relationships or motherhood itself in terms of unresolved
family issues.

The serial relationships of these women coincide with an
increasing general trend toward serial monogamy versus a lifetime
commitment. From this perspective, serial relationships appear to
be less of a thorny psychological or developmental issue and more
of a sociological one. In addition, because women commonly
develop themselves through relationships, it is not surprising that
serial relationships would be a pattern as they try to sort out their
needs and desires regarding such an important issue as motherhood.

A complication that transitional women face in resolving their
maternal ambivalence is that effective birth control has also given
men the option of deciding whether they really want to have a child.
Not only do coupled transitional women have to process their own
ambivalence about parenthood, they must sometimes deal with
their mate's ambivalence as well. Because women's ability to bear a
child is time-limited by their "biological clocks," whereas men have
no such biological restriction, the decision to have a child may, for
the woman, be decided by the passage of time before the man has
resolved his own ambivalence. In relationships where the woman is
older than her mate, which in recent years has become more
common and socially acceptable, this is more likely to happen. The
choice of a younger man comes with very real opportunity costs.
One woman at age 38 married a man several years younger. She
found that:

> A year and a half into the marriage it was disconcerting to
> discover that he didn't want children any time soon. So we've
> talked about [the fact] that his not being ready may mean that
> the biological clock runs out for me. And he just really doesn't
> feel ready at all. I don't feel, and I'll have to do some

psychological work around this, I don't feel so strongly that I would end my marriage with my husband to go meet somebody that really wanted to have a child quickly.

Transitional Women and Creative Labors

My work is very important in my life. It has been a spiritual journey of sorts.

Fifteen of the transitional women were professionals, eleven were nonprofessionals, three were students, and two were unemployed. These women are more mixed about the meaning of work for their lives. For all of them, becoming a mother was assumed to be a part of their unfolding agenda. As some of these women see their childbearing years fading, they realize that their work has indeed been more central to their identity than they could acknowledge previously. Like the women who choose not to become mothers, their work is a significant vehicle of creative expression, but they have not been as conscious of its importance as were the transformative women. One 41-year-old woman, married for many years, began in our interview to realize that her career evolution from medical technology to counseling psychology had been more than just finding the right job; she started to view it as a highly meaningful personal journey: "All these years I've been nurturing my career. It seems like my career has been my child." For these women the critical importance of their nonmaternal work as a satisfying arena for creative play is rarely present from the beginning, as it is for many transformative women. The realization seems to gradually dawn on them.

Often several job changes or a return to school for advanced education is necessary before work assumes a defining and anchoring function for these women's identities. This fluctuation may be related to a strongly held unconscious assumption of motherhood as a necessary component of their self-fulfillment. Among some transitional women their work evolves into a creative labor only in tandem with the receding possibilities of motherhood. In this pattern a woman starts a job or career path but finds it doesn't really satisfy her. She then abandons this work, holding in her mind the idea that she doesn't really need her work to be a creative labor because she plans to have a family, which will be her *real* creative work. As time passes and childbearing is increasingly less probable (or impossible by virtue of infertility) she begins to realize her life will not be as expected. The creative energy "reserved" for motherhood must be redirected; the alternative is to view herself as incomplete, defective, a failure—many women faced with this prospect and deeply tied to the unitary concept of self-fulfillment through motherhood reinforced by their external environment do indeed continue to perceive themselves in these terms. At this point the transitional woman must reorganize her sense of self toward developing and investing in her work as a creative endeavor.

This reorientation can result in a change of work, but not necessarily. Work that has not been viewed as a creative expression up to this point may become so when a woman successfully shifts from an adult identity in which motherhood is a major (if potential) component to an adult identity that does not include motherhood. This internal shift is critical; the specific nature of the work is not. A woman may expand or deepen her present work, professional or nonprofessional, by permitting it to engage her creative self. One 46-year-old women who had wanted children but found that relationship circumstances never came together in a way she wanted reoriented herself to her job. Instead of working full-time, she took a part-time legal secretary position in which she could put more of herself into both the work and the people, and began taking courses in interior design with an eye toward developing a consulting business in the future.

She may change jobs as part of this process, or she may return to school to develop a new, more potentially satisfying capacity. June, the 42-year-old woman described in this chapter, abandoned a dissatisfying teaching job in her mid-20s. A period of self-exploration followed, accompanied by a number of part-time jobs. When, in her early 30s, she realized that time would soon eclipse her chances for a family, she returned to graduate school and took a degree in public health. Now she notes that "work is a major piece of my identity," a comment she clearly would not have made 10 years earlier.

Though we have generally spoken here of formal work in the sense of employment, the concept of "work" must not be defined too narrowly. A woman may take on a specific creative project that somehow feels connected to her inner sense of self. One 45-year-old woman who was already in a satisfying profession, emphasized the importance of her own personal writing as part of her creative play when she said: "My poetry started as a way to express a wound, and now it has become a way to explore life." Writing projects, art work, dance, volunteer and community work, or nurturing specific relationships (i.e., nieces and nephews, etc.) are all endeavors that can embody and express the creative energy of a woman. That these arenas are often considered less meaningful avenues of personal identity development is less a statement of reality than it is a confusion of economic meaning with personal meaning.

The women who actively decide to to remain childless ("transformative" women) actively choose their work, together with other aspects of their lives, as satisfying their needs to develop personal identity. Transitional women, on the other hand, are confronted with the need to redefine themselves and seek nonmaternal expressions of their creativity. When faced with the reality that motherhood will not be part of their lives (either biologically or through adoption), they must relinquish this aspect of their personal identities and expand other aspects (their work or additional creative activities) to fulfill of those parts of themselves that had been held in reserve for motherhood.

Karen

I am a "transition woman." There's a part of me, a very deep and fundamental part of me that says I am to be taken care of. But when I have to be out there on my own instincts, they are pretty good. I can survive. But I haven't prospered, and the reason I haven't prospered is because I've been so busy finding the next boyfriend or husband to take care of me that I hadn't stopped long enough to reinvest in myself as an entity.

Karen, the middle child in a family of three sisters, is a 42-year-old divorced African-American woman. Her mother was divorced and dating Karen's father when she became pregnant. Although Karen's parents did not marry, her father acknowledged Karen as his child within their community, and he fulfilled the role of a divorced father in many respects even after her mother remarried when Karen was four:

> *Culturally, it was a big thing for a man who was not married to a woman to acknowledge his children. Not to say men didn't acknowledge their children; of course they did. But what I'm saying is that it was a point of pride for that woman and the child, because even though they might not have gotten married there was a family unit created that was acknowledged by all people involved. So there the marital aspects of being together were not so much the issue. The acceptance, acknowledgment, and validation of the child and the status of the child was really the issue. So the fact that my father was around, that he was a businessman, that I could go to the barber shop, I got allowance, I knew his friends, they knew I was his daughter — all of those things were very important in the parenting process. The fact that my mother and father talked about me on the telephone, etcetera. I knew that was happening.*

In Karen's first four years of life her mother worked as a seamstress and her much older sister returned home to care for her. When she remarried, Karen's mother quit work to become a homemaker. When she and Karen's stepfather divorced nine years later, Karen's mother returned to work, and later went back to school and became a social worker. Karen's experiences in early childhood, seeing her mother's difficulty in "providing," convinced her that single parenting was not what she wanted for herself:

> *When I was about twelve the beginnings of my own sense of being a mother came into being. It was realizing sexual consequences—that babies were made that way.*

[When you made the connection about sex and babies, what were your feelings about it?]

> *I was traumatized, because it meant that for the first time I had to come to grips with my repeating the pattern of my mother and father. . . . In other words, I had to deal with what that process was about. . . . My father agreed to take care of me in terms of support, but he was not going to get married to my*

mother. This has played a very heavy part in my life in the concept of motherhood. At the same time that I became aware of perhaps being a mother, it was also glaring as to how I was going to do it. Was I going to do it the way they had done it? What were my options? Was I going to find Prince Charming and be taken away to be married before I have a baby?

Karen's childhood bridged two economic worlds and two different value systems: working class and middle class. Her stepfather was a member of the working class, but her father was a middle-class businessman, and his status affected her thinking about having a child:

> *For a middle-class black woman or girl, whether she was economically middle class or value-wise middle class, welfare was unheard of. There was no option there whatsoever. You'd slash your wrists before you'd go on welfare. I don't know how representative I am of the type, but there's a bind there. The bind is that you are not lower-class enough to find welfare tenable, but [by] the same token you aren't upper class enough economically to have a safety net under you if something [pregnancy] should happen. So you opt out, or you try and wait until you can put that net under you; but you have to put that net under yourself.*

Having experienced the economic hardship of supporting a child and being unmarried, Karen's mother expressed fears about her daughter becoming pregnant outside of marriage. For this reason, among others, Karen spent a great deal of time on her urban neighborhood streets, forming significant relationships with adults who took a parental or mentoring interest in her and helped her develop the skills needed to survive in the world—skills that her mother seemingly had not had available. These "street smarts," as she called them, became integrated with her mother's value of "dignity and pride" in oneself as Karen was poised to begin adult life.

At 18 Karen married her childhood sweetheart, who was in the military. The marriage lasted two years, and she had not seriously considered having a child with this man. This early marriage seems to have been an expression of the psychic importance of a sense of stability in her life.

Shortly after the divorce Karen married her second husband, John. She was in this relationship for four years. In this second marriage Karen notes she "got the first inkling of the split between making babies and making money." John wanted to start a business, and enlisted her work experience as an employment counselor to provide needed information and contacts in the business community. During this venture she realized the tremendous energy and time commitment demanded by a creative enterprise, and developed the sense that being a mother *and* launching a business would have been impossible. This marriage ended because the couple experienced increasing conflict regarding their different views of success and financial security. At this point in her life Karen was unable to see that her own wishes for success were being expressed as expectations of how successful her husband should be.

Between the ages of 25 and 35 Karen had several relationships with men who were, in one way or another, unavailable. Although satisfactory for her in some ways, none of the relationships were with men she considered "father material" (age difference, man didn't want children, economic instability, etc.). As she discussed this period of her life, she realized that she had taken some real chances. At times she would not use birth control, at one level wishing to become pregnant and at the same time terrified that she would. In a couple of relationships she tested the level of her partner's commitment by implying she might be pregnant, with poor results. From the vantage point of being 42, Karen was able to see that she had been working out some of her issues with her father and stepfather:

> I wasn't doing it [playing Russian roulette with birth control and testing her relationships] from—well, let me back up here. I was going to say I wasn't doing it from a vindictive perspective as much as trying to get information. But I'm equally sure now that there was a substantial amount of rage and anger underneath it, but I've only been able to get to that and understand it in the last five years.

Karen did become pregnant at about the time she returned college at 32. This pregnancy may have expressed the positive side of her maternal ambivalence, or her fears of becoming more assertive/successful than she was yet ready to deal with. It may have been an expression of both. She aborted this pregnancy, giving as her reason "I was secure enough to [risk a relationship] knowing that there was the option of getting out because, as a single woman, I could get out. But I would not have felt comfortable enough to put myself and a child at risk." Her explanation represents the experience of almost two-thirds of the women interviewed who had had abortions. It was not the absence of a desire for a child that determined the decision, but, rather, not wanting a child given the current conditions of her life and relationship.

Karen married Ken at 35. The marriage lasted five years, but the business partnership they developed has continued to the present.

Each of Karen's marriages ended due to an incongruity of expectations, often the unconscious expectations of both partners. Frequently this incongruity revolved around the level of worldly success the man intended to achieve. In retrospect, Karen could see that she had selected men with "potential," men through whom she attempted to act out her own desires for involvement in the world. Karen experienced a form of inner conflict typical of the transitional woman. She thought she should be taken care of by a man, and could not acknowledge her own interests and drives. She therefore did everything she could to promote the success of her men:

> I believe in my heart that there is an entire group of women who grew up in the old school who were the women behind the men; but, man, that poor guy, he better not turn the engine off, because she was in there pumping. And she was getting her satisfaction through him, because there was no other place for her to channel it. Needless to say that, although many men were drawn to me because of my strength, it was also the same reason they wanted to get out of there; because it was too tight.

By working hard to further her husband's success so he could fulfill her myth of Prince Charming, her own "street smarts," her own accumulating job skills and talents, and her own education were channeled into his career. By the end of her third marriage, Karen realized that this pattern had kept her from truly investing in herself. Like it or not, she was actually living out her version of the "Cinderella complex." From this last marriage she learned to claim her own wishes for a creative enterprise, and to separate a business relationship from a marital one. As a result of this differentiation, she has been able to maintain both a business relationship and a friendship with Ken, her last husband.

As her third marriage was ending Karen, now 40, returned to the university to pursue a career of her own, in addition to the joint business venture. This new career is intended to combine her "savvy" with her interest in proliferating reproductive technologies and organ transplants, as well as to capitalize on her prior media and marketing experience.

> Basically what I'm doing is tracking how reproductive technology is diffused into the popular culture through the media. How does the media make what was once esoteric and not on the lips of anyone except a few doctors—how has that gone into the popular culture to turn in vitro fertilization, for instance, into a business? How is it marketed? What mythological things are touched or manipulated in order to market these services, etcetera?

At this point in her life, the issues of economic and psychic vulnerability related to having a child alone have dissipated. Having a child is no longer pressing. She realizes now that much of her delay in having a child was because she needed "to come to grips with [her] own 'woman power'"—her own strength and competency—characteristics often labeled as masculine. Karen's fear of being labelled masculine accentuated her difficulties in intimate relationships. She repeatedly tried to channel herself through the men she was with, rather than acting on her own ambitions. She is increasingly integrating her own "woman power":

> The irony is I've always backed my husbands or boyfriends. I've always had enough marketing and street savvy that I put them out there. . . . So now what I'm getting ready to do is to put out there for me the same kind of energy and effort.

Most of Karen's friends have had children, but the fact that she has none has not been especially problematic. She attributes this in part to a lesser segmentation within the African-American community between women who are mothers and those who are not. In fact, she said:

> *I've heard how wonderful kids are, and yet every woman I have ever met who has dealt with me on the basis of my childlessness, in other words, my status versus theirs, has always said, well, it's almost a litany. It ranges from things like "Girl, you are lucky. I love my kids, but, girl, you are so lucky you don't have any."*

[Why do they say that?]

> *Because they are your kids; when you get them, they are yours. I don't care who you are with, or how much you love him, those are your babies and you got to take care of them. And I'm talking about upper-class women, middle-class women, working-class women, black women, hispanic women, white women, green women. It's the world of women. What I've heard, and this is me as a desirous mother, this is me wanting a child, this is me a business woman, this is me as analytical woman, [what I've heard] is the waking up that occurs when the baby is there and is hungry, or needs changing, or has to go get some shoes, and the list goes on. While I know these children are enjoyed by these women, I also have been privy to the fact that my status as a childless woman is sometimes enviable.*

In speaking of female friendship, Karen voiced the common conflicting priorities and loyalties of minority women concerning the women's movement. Karen struggled with feelings that she would be betraying African-American men if she aligned by gender and not by race; that perhaps she would be unwittingly participating in a white man's patriarchal plan to bring white women into the labor market (at lower wages, no doubt) in an effort to exclude minority men. Like many transitional women, Karen was involved in the political movements of the 1960s, particularly the civil rights movement. Her mixed feelings regarding the women's movement abated over time, because the abortion issue has clarified the meaning of gender as an issue, and because feminism has matured in its recognition of women's ethnic differences.

Now we're [black women] in real good company again. Where the lessening of the pain comes from is that we as black women look around us. We see that hispanic women aren't getting it, white women aren't getting it. At that point, there's almost a relief to recognize that, as women, we're all in this. It isn't race; it's gender.

Of her present life, Karen says that for "the first time [her] plans aren't contingent upon what a man is going to do." She no longer perceives her strength and competence as "masculine" and has shifted from overcontrolling it to accepting it and allowing it to empower her.

In addition, Karen has been "moving toward connecting with the feminine." This has included expanding her relationships with women to include greater depth and dimensions of intimacy, especially concerning creative labors other than childrearing. She is in the process of evolving a stance in the world that accesses and utilizes both her "masculine" and "feminine" aspects. She has shifted from trying to fit in, to

believing that reality occurs because it is consensual. I believe reality occurs because you think it, and you can move on it, and you can harness the resources to make it happen. I am now not a believer that this is the way the world is and I have to somehow conform and fit in it. My belief is, this is the way the world is now, so what do I have to do to make it fit into what I have to do?

In a position she calls being "world mother," Karen plans to develop her career and establish relationships with younger women to mentor and nurture. At the present time she has a "world mother" relationship with Mary, a 21-year-old Latina woman. Karen is both confidante and home base for this young woman, in addition to being a mentor, that is, helping Mary define and move toward her career goals while in college. Karen has found an alternative role for her maternal desire.

Karen's family history made her both exceedingly self-reliant and uncertain of male reliability. Her cultural epoch provided expanding opportunities for minorities and women. These combined synergistically, creating circumstances that caused her to delay, and ultimately forego, childbearing. Like a number of transitional women, Karen's struggle to operationalize what she refers to as her masculine and feminine selves expresses the difficulty women can have in acknowledging, acting on, and giving meaning to the broad range of a woman's desires beyond motherhood. For transitional women like Karen, the path of becoming women who are not mothers involves integrating their duality of desire (which they often see as divided into female and male categories) into a cohesive adult female identity that somehow satisfies both desires.

> *I've been split because, historically, I have seen my woman self looking for Prince Charming. I have also seen my male self kicking the world in the ass to a certain extent. It has only been in the last couple of years that I have seen that split and begun to integrate the two selves. So now I empower my woman self to do what I have allowed my male self to do, and I soften my male self to allow myself to "schmooz" through situations and not attack [them] with brute force. That is an integration process of selves that I've had to do. Now I'm getting to the point where I see they don't have to be so separate.*

June

June, a petite 42-year-old Anglo-American, with a delightful sense of humor matching her elflike appearance, was interviewed at my office. She began the interview by saying:

> *I don't remember too much about my early thoughts about motherhood except assuming I would have children.*

[And why did you assume that?]

> *Probably [from] parents, people around me. I grew up in the Midwest. People thought you grew up, went to college, and had children. It was kind of expected. So I thought I'd probably do that, too.*

June is the middle child in a family of three daughters, each born two years apart. Her parents were in their late 30s and 40s when they began to have children, which was unusual for their generation. Perhaps as a result of this delay they "took parenting seriously" as well as seeming to enjoy it. Her mother and father assumed traditional roles—mother was a homemaker and father provided for the middle-class family.

As the middle child June did not see herself as having any particular role in the family apart from her being the most physically active daughter. The value her parents placed on education and achievement manifests itself in her own life. June describes her relationship with both parents as positive in temperament and interests, but she described herself as more like her father, about whom she said:

> He was a little more accepting of my doing different things. He didn't get married till thirty-nine. I remember thinking in my thirties, "I'm kind of like my dad." When he was going through that younger period he explored . . . did a number of interesting things and married late. So in some ways I thought maybe my path is sort of like his.

In light of the fact that her parents had had children late in life, I asked June what messages she had received from her parents regarding her having children.

> In my thirties my dad was especially concerned about it, and he would give me advice about the type of men I should meet. . . . When I got in my later thirties he said, "You should marry a widower who has a couple of kids, because I think it wouldn't be too safe for you to have children now." He definitely was thinking about the issue. He followed all along, and at that point he had to revise his thought a little bit. So he was always invested in it. My mother was more philosophical about it. She said, "Maybe you'll always be single, but you'll always have your friends."

June's comments conveyed a sense that her mother, however much she enjoyed being a parent herself, could see her daughter as a separate person, someone who was potentially on a different life path. Both of June's sisters had children. This raises the possibility that June is the daughter who identifies consciously with her father's adventurous nature and unconsciously carries the part of her mother that could have enjoyed the freedom of remaining single.

Like approximately a third of the women with whom I spoke, June had a significant woman in her early life who did not have children and who left a positive mark on her development:

> *My great aunt . . . was single and kind of a character. She was a professor of speech. She was always an individual. I always enjoyed talking to her when I was young, because she was one of the few people who would cut through all of the small talk and find out where I was in my life—what I was doing and what I was feeling about things. That was nice, to have a strong single woman to identify with. She was the strongest other family member for me. She was not afraid to lead her own life.*

After completing her undergraduate work, June had her first confrontation with potential motherhood when she became pregnant from her very first sexual experience at the age of 21. I asked her about the experience of being pregnant and deciding to have an abortion:

> *It was easy to know that it wasn't the appropriate time. I was in graduate school. I was with a man I didn't want to have a lasting relationship with. So, I mean, I didn't want to have a child. But at that time it was traumatic; abortions were illegal. There was a lot of anxiety in trying to get the abortion set up. It was a secret, and you had to go out of state. It was negative, definitely, for years. Of course my parents never knew about it. I couldn't even mention it to [a friend] without crying.*

The experience made her directly confront her sexuality, its consequences, and family values. The abortion experience and the social milieu of the late 1960s contributed to what June calls her "drop-out" phase, which lasted from the age of 23 to 30:

> *In my twenties I did break out of the mold, and I had a hippie drop-out phase in which I wasn't in a primary relationship but*

*was trying out a lot of different types of relationships and
different lifestyles; then I didn't even think of having children.*

[And so all during this time it sounds like you were exploring
other parts of yourself.]

*Yeah, [parts] that I hadn't had a chance to because I was always
on the very straight and narrow path. . . . I wanted to see what
else there is.*

During these years, which spanned the late 1960s and early '70s,
June followed a path common for many women and men of her age
group. Though not particularly politically active, she moved from
the Midwest to the San Francisco Bay Area, certainly one of the
cultural centers of the time. After teaching for a year in Berkeley she
quit her job in dissatisfaction and began a period of taking odd jobs
to support herself; she also moved closer to the ocean. June became
involved with the "spiritual end of things," taking various classes in
yoga and massage, experimenting with drugs, and spending a lot of
time being in nature and exploring different relationships. At the
age of 30 another psychic shift occurred:

*At thirty I went traveling for seven months and came back
really feeling, "OK, now my extended adolescence is over." I
was ready for a good relationship and to see again what I
wanted to do with career. When I came back I met a man that I
had a relationship with for six years. During that time I would
periodically bring up, hypothetically, to him that if I wanted to
have children I ought to have them pretty soon, and he would
always say, "I'm not ready for that commitment." . . . I was in
that relation from thirty-one to thirty-seven, so when that
ended I kind of went, "Oh, here I am in my late thirties and
don't have children and I don't have a primary relationship." I
guess it was at that time I had to do a little thinking about it, and
I felt I hadn't done as much as a lot of people. One way I . . . I
was going to say, rationalized, or thought about it was that I
decided that if I could have one or the other—children or a
career—I'd probably find a career more rewarding throughout
life. Now I know that it doesn't have to be [an] either/or
situation, but at that point in my life that is how I decided to*

look at it. So then I went back to school, and at age forty got my second master's degree in a field I thought I would enjoy.

[Did it seem to you at that point when you realized the relationship had ended that the time frame (for having children) had collapsed on you?]

Yes, because up until then, when I was in the relationship, I thought it still might work out.

So, at 38, another psychic shift occurred. June's assumption about having children was no longer tenable when she realized she had arrived into her late 30s without being in a committed relationship. At this point in her life, no doubt somewhat bruised by her relationship breakup, June decided to devote her energy to seriously developing a creative endeavor, rather than banking on finding and building a relationship quickly enough to have a child of her own:

It wasn't completely an active decision, as if I had stood up more for my needs in my thirties and could have foreseen that this relationship would have ended, and left in two years instead of six years. But I'm also, I'm not totally devastated by not having children.

In this statement June acknowledges her own maternal ambivalence. Previously she had let the negative part of the ambivalence be carried by a man who had indicated his own reluctance to make a commitment to marriage or children.

After her relationship broke up she returned to graduate school to get a degree in a health field. I asked her to describe her work in terms its place in her current life, and whether there were other pieces of her that carry important aspects of her sense of identity:

I think right now work is the major one. I think this partly goes along with not having a primary relationship.

June makes it clear here that, although her work is now a central aspect of her identity in a way that it certainly was not in her 20s, a primary relationship would be of equal importance in defining her sense of self, were she to have one. In our follow-up interview, June indicated she had been in a relationship for the last year. Her partner is a number of years younger than she; and early in the relationship she brought up the issue of her being too old to have children, indicating the consolidation of her identity as a woman who does not intend to become a mother.

> *I asked him early on in our relationship about his ideas about having children and how he felt about choosing to be with a woman who is too old to have them.*

While she has established a field for her creative labor, her goals are still developing. June is leaving space for the primary relationship she has entered to have an influence upon certain of her long-range plans.

At the time of the initial interview June was moving from one part of the Bay Area to another, and reestablishing a support system. Now, a few years later, she has a number of women friends who are also without children. At this point, she surveys her peers and takes in both the reality of her own childlessness and the life option it represents:

> *Seeing couples who have decided not to have children has made me feel somewhat better. It's like, "Well, here are people who are in a good relationship and are deciding not to have children." It makes me less odd in my not having children. It also kind of surprises me; I don't know why. I guess that's the traditional conditioning—married people have children. But I'm glad to know there are alternatives; that married people can choose not to have children.*

She is shifting her perspective about what not having children means. Parenting is no longer an expected result of every marriage, but one expression of a direction that marriage may take. Whereas in the past more of her friends had children, in recent years more do not—this development of different relationships is part of her transition into a female identity that does not include motherhood in its definition. There is a sense that June has less acceptance of the stigma attached to childlessness, which was a residue of her Midwestern "straight and narrow path." I asked her: "If you think about the issue that most women are mothers and this is a central part of who they are, what thoughts do you have about being a woman who doesn't have kids, and what sort of reactions have you gotten?" She replied:

> *That is interesting, this does happen. There is a new nutritionist starting on one of the projects who asked me if I had children. And I said "no," and I know when I say that I always feel a little bad about saying "No, I don't have children."*

[And the feeling bad comes from?]

> *Well, it's true I don't know. There's two parts: Am I feeling bad because it's something I really wanted and don't have?; or Is it feeling bad because it is something other people have and I always have to say I don't? I just don't know.*

[Is there anything about this issue of having children that you would redo?]

> *That whole period in my twenties; if I could have shortened that a little bit. It seems like maybe I take a little long in each of my phases to go through it; if that could have been shortened. I certainly wasn't ready to have children until I was in my thirtiess to mid-thirties. It is hard to see how I could have done things differently. The men who wanted to have a lasting relationship were in college . . . but I wasn't ready at that time. It seems partly timing and not meeting the right person at the right time. I wasn't yet ready when I was younger, and then when I was somewhat older the right relationship didn't develop.*

When asked about the most significant influences of the past 20 years for shaping her present adult identity it is not surprising that June mentioned the 6-year relationship she had in her 30s, both in its positive and negative aspects. She also remarked that "Going back to school finally and taking a little more control of my life to get into a field of work where I have a marketable skill and enjoy my work was a major positive step." By ending the relationship rather than continuing to drift in it, and then by returning to school, June was shifting her subjective position in relation to her life from "going with the flow" on the question of motherhood and her life to a more active position of interpreting her desires and making plans to act on them. The decision to return to school was the birth of herself as a women who is not a mother. It also represented a move toward opening the void created by the loss of imagined children to other offspring that might emerge from inside her. June's movement toward accepting the loss of motherhood by returning to school rather than engaging in an all-out effort to find another relationship represents the necessary step childless women must take to symbolically "hold" the emptiness of their physical wombs receptive to other kinds of "offspring" emerging from this symbolic space.

June's response to my query asking her to imagine her life from the perspective of herself as an elder woman reflected the androgynous orientation many transitional women seek. She said she wanted to have had a life that balanced satisfying work with her connections with people. In saying "I would like to see it as an interesting life, and a little unconventional," her primary sense of self seems to encompass those features of her family members and the social values of her youth that, together with a certain amount of fate, combined to place her on an atypical pathway of adult female development.

Conclusion

It is tempting to look at the maternal ambivalence as expressed in the lives of "transitional" women from a traditional gender role perspective and to conclude that the ambivalence results from unresolved family issues. Yet to do so would be to pathologize this entire pathway of adult female identity. This would be analogous to assuming there is "psychological health" among all those adults who have children. The sociological changes of the last decades have opened new spaces for women (and men) to move into. Sometimes, in doing so, other spaces are left empty; other identity possibilities, specifically in the case of transitional women the possibility of motherhood, are left unexplored.

Because motherhood has historically been so central to female identity, sooner or later the transitional woman must address its absence in her life, and must assess what, if anything, is "missing." She must shift from a position of "going with the flow" of her life, with motherhood assumed to be part of her future, to wondering what it means that motherhood is indeed missing. Addressing the notion of absence, or "something missing," is a necessary part of affirming her atypical female identity. When motherhood is no longer possible, women like June discover that their work shifts from being only a job to becoming a creative endeavor. In so doing they find that the "something missing" does not leave as big a void as had been expected. Other women find there is really nothing "absent," and, as it is for many men, life is fulfilling without parenthood. Others, like Karen, who had stronger maternal inclinations, redirect their maternal feelings into alternative maternal roles, similar to the process of some traditional women.

So long as the transitional woman remains in a state of unconsciousness regarding her child*less* or child-free circumstances, the process of defining and claiming her own life will be inhibited. A woman must shift from the subjective position of "being in" the experience of being "child*less* or child-free" to a subjective position of wondering how she got there and interpreting what this may mean to her identity. Karen needed to confront the fact that her inability to find a relationship that ever felt suitable for having a child was partly the result of not having "owned" her ambition to be in the world in a nonmaternal way. June clearly experienced some regret that her childless circumstances were partially a result of her needing a prolonged period of exploration in order to grow into herself. For June this developmental pathway had mixed consequences. It provided her with a diversity of experiences (as a similar path had done for her father), but it inhibited her development of a relationship in which to have a child (as her mother had). When faced with her impending childlessness, June shifted her maternal ambivalence in the direction of developing her career (rather than expending a final, all-out effort to quickly find a relationship in which to try and have a child) and discovered her loss was less than she had anticipated it would be.

As the transitional woman in a heterosexual relationship realizes she and her partner will not be parents together, she must revise her expectations and discover other points of connection with men. Karen realized she had to accept as her own the parts of herself (her desires for a career) that she had given to her partners and then expected them to live out for her.[5] When she was able to shift her expectations and allow more of herself to be empowered, her relationships with men changed. By reaching a deeper understanding regarding her own contributions to their marital difficulties, Karen was able to maintain a business and friendship relationship with her ex-husband.

When she was able to confront the reality that her expectations for marriage and family were not going to be met, June was able to break off a 6-year relationship. As she realized motherhood was not to be part of her life, her expectations of men as primary partners also began to change. June has found she is now more able to permit whatever relationship she develops to take its own unique form.

Transitional women whose creative energies are successfully channeled into work or other endeavors meaningful to them experience greater satisfaction with their lives and more personal comfort with their "different" status in society. They are less likely to accept society's view of them as "deviant" or "incomplete." For women like Karen there is often an process whereby characteristics previously conceived of as "male" are integrated into a more complete concept of "female," thereby consolidating a personal identity independent of societal gender role expectations.[6]

Some women, like June, require less of an integrative process, having developed their atypical female identities through identifications with mothers and/or significant women in their past. June's identification with her childless great aunt enabled her to act on her desire for creative work and yet still feel connected to a "female" sense of self.

When a woman can acknowledge that she will not be a mother and can begin to accept the loss of that pathway to adult female identity, she can utilize other creative endeavors to affirm a positive nonmaternal adult female identity. Creative and nurturing energies are not "missing" from women who are not mothers, but they are not expressed through the bearing and raising of children. When there is no awakening consciousness, a woman's creative endeavors may remain another "piece" of her identity rather than serving as an element to organize her identity and direct its expression. Left unconscious, the potential identity as mother will remain within her self-concept, reminding her that something isn't altogether congruent in her life—an unhealed and unhealable bruise. When this psychic bruise is "bumped" (as it can be when others ask "Do you have children?") the issue of maternity will be uncomfortably revived. Yet, each of these bruising encounters also provides an opportunity for the process of resolution to begin.

The traditional woman illustrates most clearly the primary dynamic of mourning of a lost opportunity in order to develop the adult female identity, because maternity was integral to her sense of who she would become. The transitional woman illustrates the tension and conflict of multiple desires and the dialectical process of shifting between subjective positions with regard to one's life. (The mourning of the transitional woman will be variable, depending on the extent to which the potential identity of mother was a part of her unique, unconscious, personal identity.)

The transitional woman illustrates a dimension of struggle and sacrifice. Struggling to reconcile and fulfill both maternal and nonmaternal desires, and faced with the reality that childbearing is no longer possible, she may consciously accept her own particular child*less* circumstances, letting go of her identification with her womb as the place to nourish a child so that another kind of creative child may be born. In this act of conscious letting go, a different path is opened. An inability to relinquish the (for her) unrealizable aspect of motherhood for the sake of something else, something often unknown, can result in a life pervaded by bitterness, disappointment, and a sense of failure.

As transitional women faced with the realization that childbearing was not to be part of their lives, Karen and June were eventually able to release those aspects of their potential adult identities revolving around motherhood in order to be open to whatever else could be born from the space within.

4

The Transformative Woman: Child-free

I can't remember if I ever thought I had a choice. I think I
thought you just did it. You grow up and you have children.
. . . There came a time when I was thirty-five. It was really
obvious, despite my fantasies and making up stories, that I
don't really want [a child] or I would have been out there
having one. And I wanted to be a socially responsible person,
so I had my tubes tied.

Unlike the "traditional" or "transitional" woman, the "transformative" woman chooses a child-free life and places herself on a
little-traveled path. She is essentially a trailblazer, creating a path
through a thicket of meanings of what a woman "should be" and
yet often isn't.

There is more resistance to recognizing the female identity of
the transformative woman. She is more likely to have organized her
identity around autonomy; because of this she can be judged by
others as having a "masculinity complex." Consider the common
stereotype of the childless woman as "that hard-driving career
woman." It is not surprising that these women tend to remain
"invisible" in discussions of adult development, because their
presence challenges many unconsciously accepted preconceptions
of what women "should be." The categorization of characteristics
into female and male attributes poses problems. Women and men
both become restricted in the human characteristics they may
identify with or act on without being labeled deviant.

Transformative women endorse characteristics of independence such as assertiveness and leadership capacity—traits more commonly associated with the traditional male sex role. Research has shown that women identifying with characteristics of a masculine sex role have higher self-esteem and sense of competency than do women who identify with those traits associated with the stereotypical feminine sex role.[1] The transformative woman is thus more able than either the traditional or transitional woman to deflect negative social judgments about her child-free life. With a greater sense of self-confidence she is more likely to respond to such judgements with her own query as to why a woman's life must be bounded by the institution of motherhood.

When the transformative woman chooses to remain child-free, she is saying to the world that she is on a personal quest in which motherhood plays no part. She is making a conscious decision to explore other avenues of expression for whatever maternal feelings she has. Whatever her life choices, the transformative woman needs to experience internal affirmation, because she lives in a world that is not yet comfortable with her atypical female identity. Others may question not only her judgment in choosing not to have children, but the very foundation of her feminine being.

The transformative woman's life illustrates most clearly that a nonparental creative life can be a focus for a woman as much as it can be for a man. She has made a conscious choice to develop her identity in nonmaternal creative labor.

For transformative women the cultural context of feminism provided a feeling of legitimacy and value. For the first time, they didn't have to feel *deviant*. A 39-year-old transformative woman whose mother and grandmother were not enthusiastic mothers was able to decide to attend medical school rather than continue a legacy of unenthusiastic motherhood. Regarding the influence of feminism on her decision, she felt "there was a place for me, and I was able to be authentic and as true to myself and what I believe in as any human being has had a chance to." Her mother had once said to her: "I never wanted to have children. Of course you feel differently about your own, but I never particularly wanted to have children." The importance of the interrelation of family background and historical times is clear in this woman's response:

> I think either explicitly or implicitly the message I got from all
> the women in the family was they didn't like it [motherhood]—
> it wasn't appealing. The difference between me and them was
> the message wasn't new to my generation. I'm sure my mother
> must have gotten the same message from her mother and
> grandmother, but somehow, someway, I didn't do it.

This "somehow and someway" was due to the general ethos of the
1960s and of feminism in particular, which said "you don't *have* to
do it."

Transformative Women and Primary Relationships

> I've always thought I would make a good "father" because I
> enjoy children, but I've never wanted to be the "primary
> parent." And most men do not want to be the primary parent,
> either.

The relationship pattern of transformative women is strikingly
different from that of traditional women. Because these women do
not want to fulfill a traditional role of mother, they seek out a
different kind of man and relationship. Among the 39 transformative women I spoke with, fourteen were married, eight were living
with a partner or in a committed relationship (five of these were
heterosexual and three were lesbian), and sixteen were single.
Twelve woman had been previously divorced; eight of these are
now in committed relationships and four are single.

There were more minority women in the transformative group
in committed relationships (75%) than in the other two groups.
Sixty-seven percent of traditional minority women were in relationships, and 40% of the transitional minority women. Since racial
minorities often experience more social pressure to become mothers
from their own subculture, the fact that these women in primary
relationships could choose not to have children suggests that
childbearing decisions are more a matter of gender than of race or
class.

The expressed intention of a man to "really" be involved in the
day-to-day caretaking of a child notwithstanding, it is many

women's conviction that the bulk of the parenting responsibility for a child will be theirs. This was the attitude of many of the transformative women. They did not want to be trapped in a culturally assigned role that they believed would preclude other activities and relationships.

One 43-year-old woman asked her husband directly: "Could you be the primary caretaker? Could you be that committed and that devoted?" When he said: "No, I think I could be a father but not a mother," she replied, "Well, I think we have two fathers in this relationship, so I think it [having a child] isn't going to happen."

Transformative women approach or develop their love relationships with different expectations, because a child is not necessarily anticipated. Marilyn, the 39-year-old woman discussed later in this chapter said:

> There's been evolution in our relationship. I think when we first got together it was more traditional. I would do all the housework. He would do the gardening. As our relationship has evolved it's become much more a clarification of what our preferences really are. . . . Now . . . the more concrete and practical stuff [is] not based on gender. It's more based on who wants to do it, who likes to do it, or who hates it the least.

Marilyn mentioned that because she is a therapist and nurtures others all day, some evenings when she gets home she is unable to give any further. In this respect she says of her mate: "In a lot of ways he takes on a more nurturing role in relation to me."

Transformative women often express the importance of the "quality" of time spent with their partners. For some women the quality of connection to their mate was a significant factor in their decision not to have children. Exploring the world together and mutual support of each other's creative pursuits are often characteristics of their relationships. These women seemed to have sought partners with whom they could be "sojourners" through life. Another common research finding among child-free couples evident in this study was the egalitarian nature of the relationship; these women do not look to men to give them a child or provide for them in what would be considered "traditional" ways. As one 43-year-old woman described her marriage:

He puts his clothes away; I put my clothes away. It's a tremendous freedom from gender definitions as our society and family has created [them]. I'm not tied to being a traditional wife. I'm not taking care of a husband, so to speak. When I do tasks in the house I do them out of "It's my house, I like to do that or it has to get clean or this has to be bought." And he does, too. It isn't out of a role. And half the time he brings home the food for dinner.

We might think of these couples as the other side of the coin of couples who truly coparent.[2] Since the common structuring function of child raising is missing in these relationships, the paths the relationships take can vary considerably. The ambiguity and fluidity of the "structure" of these relationships is, of course, both a strength and a potential nemesis. Marilyn notes that:

We've been living apart for significant periods of time the last two and a half years. That has been a whole shifting thing, because it became a process where we had to start to go much deeper than defining who was going to do what chore. We started to define what was important to who, and how we were going to work out the fact that he wants to live in the country, while my connections and what matters to me are here. In this process I discovered I couldn't leave it all behind, so this living arrangement evolved for these couple of years. This kind of experimentation in living wouldn't have been possible if we had a child.

The potential problems in these more fluid arrangements is that there is less *external* glue or structure (which parenting provides) to hold the relationship together. Each person in the relationship must rely more on his or her own *inner* sources of identification and connection with their partners. The meaning and structure of this atypical relationship can at times feel tenuous as well as liberating—something like doing a trapeze act together without a net.

As might be expected, the relationship structure in lesbian couples is also more fluid. Although many assume that all lesbian women are transformative women, and thus choose not to have children, this is not so. In the past two decades many more lesbian woman have openly expressed their maternal desires. In past years, only those who had come to lesbianism after a marriage were mothers. This is no longer the case. One 38-year-old woman I spoke with experienced the end of a committed relationship because her partner wanted very much to have a child and she didn't want to be a coparent. Homosexual as well as heterosexual relationships have been affected by and have themselves affected decisions regarding childlessness.

Transformative Women and Creative Labors

If I weren't an artist I would have kids, but maybe a lot of the impetus to create things is satisfied in many ways by being an artist and taking nothing and making something out of it and shaping it.

Twenty-three of the transformative women were professionals, ten were nonprofessionals, two were currently in school, and three were unemployed. For many of these women their creativity is as strongly directed toward work as it is into their love relationships. In this respect their feelings about work closely parallel those society generally consider to be "male" attitudes. More than in the other two groups, these women mentioned work as one of the most significant influences of the past 20–25 years in shaping their present identities. Among these women, who decide early in adulthood to be child-free, there is the feeling that motherhood was an option they considered but did not choose, partly because they felt they could not wholly commit themselves to the task as they believed "it should be done" and simultaneously be as involved in other work as they wanted to be.

Because of the limited role of the traditional father in childcare, men generally do not experience conflict between their desires for a family and fulfillment in their work. This is, to some degree and for some men, changing, but unambivalently combining fatherhood and career remains the norm. Men generally do not view their personal success in the workplace as diminishing their success in their family role. For transformative women, however, there is an internal expectation of excellence that makes it impossible for them to pursue both creative nonmaternal work and motherhood. One 42-year-old woman whose in-laws expressed their view of her choice of childlessness as being abnormal, said: "I've always been someone who likes to focus intensely on one thing at a time and become excellent at it. I just couldn't see how I could be an excellent mother and have a career." One could speculate that the desire for excellence was not seen as abnormal; merely the alternative chosen.

Other women whose decisions to remain childless evolved over a period of time did not see work and motherhood initially as quite so mutually exclusive. Often these women select a career with the idea in mind that when they are established in that career they will then add a child to their lives.

Nonetheless, in these cases the women still end up consciously choosing a life without motherhood. They find that in the process of establishing a stable career they have found a means of satisfying their creative impulses and the desire for a child lessens in intensity. Although childbearing was maintained as a possible option, these women discovered it was not necessary to their personal identities. These women found other ways to satisfy both their needs for work and love.

Judith, the 46-year-old woman whose life is chronicled in this chapter, expected when she began studying physics that she would have children later in life. But by "following what's next" from her internal motivation, her unfolding life experience established an adult identity in which her writing incorporated her creative needs.

> I think the function of physics was to lead me through the constrictions of Newtonian reality of separate things and going all the way through causality and falling out the back door of it. . . . Photography was . . . just waiting for me. I sold a lot at student art sales, so when I decided I didn't want to be in physics I trusted I could make a living as a photographer, which turned out to be true. And then photography supported me. The next major shift was from seeing myself as a photographer to inner exploration and spirituality, and that's still ongoing. . . . I've realized what I've been learning the past few years is "cocreative work" rather than my own individual, unique creativity, or doing my own thing. [It is]how to work with somebody else. So the real learning for me is how to serve

without being servile, how to give without losing my own center. . . . I've had varying degrees of success with that—literally midwifing is the best way to put it.

A 41-year-old woman who filed a discrimination suit against a publishing house expresses the kind of energy that these women frequently embody in their lives:

I think of myself as living as fully as I can, and if that means taking a year off and wandering around Europe and writing and making as much or as little [as needed] and living on it, I'll do it.

The transformative women discussed here could be viewed from the traditional perspective as simply malcontents who are unable to accept their innate destiny as mothers. As indicated by the experiences of industrialized nations during World War II, however, what is viewed as "innately female" is actually strongly tied to cultural needs and definitions arising out of social circumstances. The appearance of transformative women in greater numbers calls for a reexamination of the notion of motherhood as central to all women's personal identity needs.

Judith

I wouldn't have been able to do what I did [photography and writing books] if I had a child or even a husband. The creative work required that I be nonfunctional at times, spending a day staring into space, waiting for something to emerge, sometimes feeling very depressed, diving into the darkness and not paying attention to anything external. Obviously I could not have done that if I had had small children. I would have been a depressed housewife, fighting it off, being neither here nor there. I would not have been able to let myself go.

Judith, a single, Anglo-American woman, was 47 years old at the time of our interview. She describes her middle-class family of origin as "the classic family: Mother, father, and two children. My mother didn't work. It was the nuclear family with all its joys and its difficulties." For a number of years in her childhood her paternal grandmother lived with them. Her maternal grandparents lived close by, so there was a strong sense of extended family in her life. As in many traditional families, her father "worked a lot" and "wasn't around that much"; yet she described her relationship with her father as involving a sense of being kindred spirits. This type of relationship seems to have also existed between her older brother and her mother.

Of the two children she was the one "who acted out, hollered, and yelled" the most. Another way she described this was that she was "feisty," like her mother.

Judith's mother and maternal grandmother were a part of a "long line of strong women" who were educated and who modeled independence within the constraints of their particular eras. Because of this heritage, Judith thought of herself as "automatically a feminist," and said she "always knew women could do things."

Judith's mother seemed to express some maternal ambivalence when she told her daughter: "Taking care of children is not all that wonderful, but you'd better do it to carry on the family line." Recently Judith visited her family and addressed this ambivalence directly:

My mother asked me, did I ever wish I had children, and I was finally able to say, "No, but I know that has not been OK with you." And she actually kind of released it and said, "Well, you know, people are different." And at that point I had accepted it myself, and it was really nice to have that acceptance mirrored to me by my mother.

[It was good to be released from this stuff with your mother because you had been afraid you were disappointing her? Or that she would feel invalidated because you were not doing the same things she did?]

Yeah. One thing that actually helped, and I think she took this in—I told her some of the work that I'd been doing was touching a lot of people, and in a way a lot of those people were her grandchildren. Of course it didn't make it totally OK, but she could sort of see that. And I dedicated a book to her, and she had loved that.

The particular blend of Judith's family history and the sociological milieu of the 1960s and 1970s produced a woman like Judith who could ultimately choose a child-free life; but she didn't start off in that direction. As did most women of her generation, Judith assumed she would have children. She anticipated childbearing only after completing her education, so she did not really think about having children during her years at the university, which extended into her late 20s.

Judith undertook graduate work in physics. The only woman in her class, she experienced firsthand the meaning of sexism and its possible impact on her scientific career. This served, in part, to deflect her from serious pursuit of a career in physics. Her growing interest in photography was also an important factor. Judith learned photography from a boyfriend while in graduate school; the field began to take on greater meaning and provided a means of real earning power after graduate school. In her first postdoctoral year she left the field of physics altogether and supported herself through photography. She also began her own path of inner exploration; her interest in physics was instrumental in developing a fascination with eastern meditation. Judith's first creative projects, utilizing her photography skills, were book collaborations with an Asian man. She was in a primary relationship with this man for 4 years and, she quipped: "We didn't have children; what we had were two books."

This primary relationship reflected the style of the times; it was a committed relationship within the context of a communal arrangement. Although never politically active (as were some of her generation) she was soon to reflect many of the ideas of the 1960s and 1970s in her lifestyle and values. In responding to a query about the forces of the past 25 years that had influenced her personal identity formation, she mentioned beginning her photographic work, some friendships, and "the whole cultural times of the 1960s that allowed the breaking of old forms and gave me the freedom to do what I have done."

In her unfolding lifestyle we see how "woman's place" began shifting within changing social paradigms. In the counterculture communal situation in which she lived, Judith consciously took on the maternal role of managing day-to-day chores and the emotional harmony of the household. At the same time she reported that whenever her mate, who was seen as a guru by some in the community, became too "patriarchal," she would walk up behind him, pick him up by the shoulders, saying "portable guru," and walk him out of the room amidst everyone's laughter. Judith saw this period as one in which she tried out her own version of the maternal role. She had realized that she did not want a "traditional life," but the question of motherhood had not yet been resolved.

Following this 4-year communal period Judy lived and worked at Esalen—a psychological "Mecca" of the 1960s. This was an intensely creative period, during which she produced another book, doing both the writing and the photography. Regarding her feelings at this time about children and childbearing she noted that:

Up until the time where I really accessed my own inner child, I really distanced myself from people with children. But since then I've enjoyed being around children. I think the shift was that being around children activated stuff in me that I was uncomfortable with, and when I befriended the internal things surrounding it, it was no longer threatening to be around children.

Following her experience at Esalen, Judith pursued the question of maternity a bit more directly by living for 3 years with a family who had one child.

When I moved in with them, they had one child about one-year-old, and by the time I moved out they had three. I was present for two home births, and did a lot of child care, changed a lot of diapers, learned how to pick up a sleeping child and put it in its bed without waking it up. And it became clear to me that I enjoyed a certain amount of contact with children, but I really did not want to the day-to-day [experience] of having one of my own. It became really clear, because experience satisfied the positive part and it also clarified the "no."

[Are you saying, Judith, that it was really a part of that experience that made it clear to you what your limits were in being in relationship with children?]

Yes, I got over some of my fears about, "Oh, I don't know how to handle children." And I realized I was quite good with children, and I also realized I didn't want to be with them full-time. There were too many other things I wanted to do.

These "other things" have not meant distancing herself from her friends with children. Approximately half of her friends have children, and these friendships have been a major source of intimacy in her life. As she puts it:

I have several families that I'm "Aunt Judith" to. [During one period, my] photographic work had a lot to do with birth-type images. They were pictures of nature. And this was during a friend's first pregnancy, [when I] was writing poetry. So we put it together in a book. In this case, the coming of the child brought us together, because I was accessing the same territory in my own internal process that she was doing through her pregnancy.

Judith's decision to remain child-free evolved over a period of years. Her relationships with others were as much a part of this evolving as was her internal process. Assuming the maternal role in her communal household and sharing childcare with a couple she lived with were two of the ways the question of motherhood cycled through her life. This is a typical pattern for the transformative woman, summarized by Judith:

Accepting and transforming childlessness has been a process. The knowing started as a kind of an intellectual acceptance, then it sank down into my heart with emotional acceptance, and finally came down into my belly; and I knew deep in my body that there were going to be no physical children coming through. In a way, the deep knowing is a great relief. There is no longer any guilt, and the creativity, the generative energies, are really fully available to go in other directions, and to parent in other ways.

Shortly after this settling of a deep-felt knowing, there was a shift in her experience of connection.

It was feeling a sense of connectedness and not being dependent on it coming through a person. It is a spiritual experience. It's just an experience of <u>connectedness</u>, not an experience of being <u>connected</u> to any particular thing.

As part of this feeling of "connectedness," she began to nurture others' creative work (particular that of other women) in addition to her own; she calls this her "midwifery." She involved herself in helping a friend select, prepare, and transport artwork for a show. This shift of Judith's to include "midwifing," or cocreative work, seems to include a recognition of the maternal aspect within herself, as well as her need to link herself through creativity to succeeding generations. She indicated that "parenting is the need to give without expecting anything in return," and there are many ways that this can occur. Although some people might ask her about the various unpaid work she does for others, she says, "but if you were a parent you'd be working without being paid for it—service is a natural thing."

Creative "midwifing" is balanced with continued pursuit of her own creative work, in the unique pattern that she has established for herself:

[So, really, since you got out of school in physics, you've been able to use that training to develop your work in such a way as to go from one project to another.]

Yeah, I just follow what's next, and then from a later perspective I can then put labels on it. At this point I would probably be incapable of holding a regular job, because I'm so used to following . . . ["your intuition?"] Yeah, my intuition, and following what's next. Not always with great confidence, sometimes letting my intuition drag me kicking and screaming into what needs to happen. And then accepting it and going through a phase of accepting it, and then into a phase of delighting in it.

The helix may be an apt image for Judith's life. Her love relationships and friendship relationships are forever interwoven with her creative endeavors. Her life has been rich in the intimacy of mentors, cocreators, and friends, and these connections have fueled her creative expressions.

There is a certain irony here because, apart from a 4-year relationship in her late 20s, Judith has not had an enduring primary relationship. She exemplifies the myth of the child-free woman as autonomous, a woman unto herself. Her move into photography represented the beginning of what was to become the signature pattern of her life—she followed a call emanating from inside herself. This has become the center of her identity, but the process of realizing that she could not respond to her internal creative voice at the level of involvement she desired and also be a mother (as the role is traditionally defined) has been a slow one. When asked how she responded to the question "Do you have children?" she replied:

> *I think I used to be sort of defensive and avoid situations like that. And now the thing that comes forth sometimes is envy from other people. Surprising how many people have children and kind of wish they didn't. That's one aspect of it. Another aspect of this is that I'm reasonably in what I am, so it isn't so much of a question of what I'm not now. In fact, that's the whole thing about the phrase "childless." The word "childless" is focusing on what you are not. So this has been another part of my own healing journey—the shift from what is not, to what is.*

The stereotype of the childless woman implies that being childless isn't so much a "real choice" as it is a reaction to having received poor mothering. Childlessness is often seen as shaped by a family history more dysfunctional than Judith's history indicates. Some transformative women's choices to remain child-free may be reactive rather than actively conscious. But a compelling impulse to bear a child can sometimes also be shaped by a dysfunctional family; it may represent an unsuccessful attempt to fill up an inner emptiness or heal old wounds.[3]

Living in a society that expects women to become mothers, a woman who does not become a mother is more immediately confronted with the need to question her own family experience. The transformative women who do come from dysfunctional families and question motherhood in terms of their family history confront a damaged childhood self—a self that needs to be healed before it feels "right" to have a child of one's own. This confrontation, and the healing it can bring, make possible a conscious decision about motherhood, rather than a reactive decision of "I just can't." In the same way, a woman confronting her background can come to truly choose to have a child, rather than making a reactive decision of "I just must."

A conscious decision to remain child-free opens a woman's life to other creative potentials in a way that a reactive decision does not. Marilyn is an example of just such a woman.

Marilyn

I've spent most of my life as a "caretaker" of others. I just wanted a chance to live life for myself. . . . I thought there must be another way [besides being a mother] to have an identity.

When I really sit down and think about it, if I give it serious thought, I always end up back on the side of not having a child. I end up on the side of living with the fear and the aloneness, and getting old, and having to cope with whatever that's going to mean. . . . I think it is exciting to decide not to have a baby, and really try to make room for your own creative self, but I also think it's really hard. I don't think it is easy. I think there are agonies involved. But I also think that there are agonies involved in being a mother, many of which are never spoken.

Marilyn is a 40-year-old Anglo-American woman who has been living with a man in a primary relationship for the past 16 years. She grew up as the oldest child in a middle-class family of five children. Marilyn's mother worked as a nursery school teacher until the birth of her third child. (When Marilyn was an adult, her mother told her that she had wanted to keep teaching but was unable to handle both work and home responsibilities.) Her father was in a business that provided the family with a stable, middle-class lifestyle; when Marilyn was about 12 her parents divorced, and his support was less predictable.[4]

Marilyn feels she received "poor parenting." She sees her mother as having been overwhelmed by the task of being the primary parent to five children and said:

I wouldn't have said this at the time, but what I would say now is that I was distant from my parents. I'd say, not truly

connected to either one of them. I can only say that now because
I feel I know what a true connection is.

She felt close to her siblings, for whom she assumed a parental role
early in life. She also mentioned an aunt as an important female
model. This woman, a working mother of three sons, was seen as
both "nurturing and competent in the world."

When Marilyn was about 10 she realized her mother had
developed an alcohol problem, which increased as her parents'
marriage worsened. About 2 years later her father left the family,
and through Marilyn's teen years provided inconsistent emotional
and financial support. Marilyn's caretaking responsibilities increased; she notes in retrospect that this early caretaker role has had
a significant bearing upon her choice not to have children. Yet at the
time Marilyn left her family to attend college, she simply assumed
that she, too, would someday marry and have several children of
her own.

During her college years Marilyn was very much involved with
the ideas, attitudes, politics, and practices of the 1960s. The Vietnam
antiwar movement was an opportunity to question the accepted
forms and values of her childhood:

I went to a very conservative Catholic [college] my first years.
Women had to wear skirts, and this kind of thing. And then that
summer between my freshman and sophomore years was that
[1968 "Summer of Love"] in the Haight-Ashbury. . . . I lived in
the Haight with two girl friends. And, boy, that was the
beginning for me. I mean, that just blew everything wide open.
. . . after I graduated I worked for the World without War
Council, and that was how I was earning a living until I started
working with the children's shelter. And then it was after, when
the women's movement was, that I got a beginning sense that it
was OK to be female. It's OK to be a woman. And I think I got
a sense that women could do things, too.

As a counselor at a halfway house for adolescents (where she
was called "Mother Marilyn" because of her dedication) she
reached a burnout point and decided to return to graduate school in
a mental health field. This was a pivotal decision in her life; it put
her on a path that utilized her caretaking skills and fulfilled

achievement needs. This return to graduate school also reflected a positive identification with her own female therapist, with whom she was exploring those parts of herself neglected during childhood years.

In her early 20s Marilyn did not think seriously about having children. As many college educated women would say, "it just wasn't an issue." In her late 20s she met her live-in partner of 16 years. At the beginning of their relationship they decided to postpone the parenting decision for 5 years in order to allow the relationship time to consolidate. After 5 years they postponed it again. It was clear to Marilyn that, from the beginning of the relationship her partner was more inclined to not have children, but he was not entirely against parenthood. She can now say that she is unsure whether their relationship would have survived conflicts over childrearing decisions and responsibilities. At present, theirs is very much an equal partnership. I asked her how having a child might have affected the nature of their relationship:

> Oh, I think it would really severely be affected. I don't think we would have nearly as much time to just do things together and be together with each other. As it is, we are both in very demanding professions. We have a dog and a cat, and sometimes dealing with them feels like more than I can deal with, much less a child. To tell you the truth, I don't know if our relationship would survive. I think it might, but I think you have to have a pretty unique kind of relationship to really successfully raise children.

[What do you see as the crucial vulnerabilities that you would be afraid would cause too much stress?]

> Oh, dear. Well, what really comes to mind is that we would fight. We would fight over how to deal with the kid. We would definitely fight over me thinking I was doing more than my share of the work with the kid. But I would be setting myself up for that. We would fight about whether we should have had this kid in the first place. I don't know, it would probably be more than that, but it would probably just stress it out. I think we would both feel deprived.

Both Marilyn and her partner prize the egalitarian nature of their life together. Her expressed concern about the loss of intimacy that parenting would exact is a common consideration of many child-free couples.[5]

Their postponement of the parenting decision shifted into active consideration as Marilyn reached her middle 30s. She saw her friends "one by one having a child" and the issue of childbearing took on greater significance for her:

> I must have gone through a spurt a few years ago when I bought a book. And I must have ended up reading close to eight or ten books on the topic through this whole process. So I went through a real conscious phase; the most intense aspects coincided with my inner development of the feminine. . . . I would go around and pretend "What would it be like to be pregnant," and stick a pillow in my nightgown and look at myself in the mirror. I think that this was really important for me because I was going through the development of my feminine side. And I think the issue of having a baby really came to the fore as part of that.

[Did you ever make the effort to get pregnant during those times? If not, why not?]

> No, not at all. I talked with my boyfriend. I did a lot of talking about it. And in some ways I was trying to convince him that maybe it would be a neat thing. Wouldn't it be cute, and that kind of stuff. But it wasn't like I was definitely decided, and really had my heart set on it. It was more like a practicing kind of thing. . . . And then it would kind of subside. And as part of this was going on I began to make a connection between the wish to have a real baby and that, in a way, this was a projection—that it was a way of making external an internal developmental process.

[And what was this process that was really on the inside that you wanted to do with this baby on the outside?]

> I think it really had to do with giving birth, or coming into my own real self. . . . I had this incredible series of dreams about

babies; having a baby, the baby getting older, the baby taking its first step, just this whole amazing maturation thing. And while I was going through all this, one of my closest friends was trying very hard to get pregnant. And she eventually did become pregnant. It raised a lot of issues for me, and I think that my friends who were pregnant or recently had children have felt kind of impatient with me, because I started getting on this little bandwagon.

[Did they think you were getting a little obsessional around this "one internal aspect" of what having a baby means?]

(Laughs) Right. They're saying, "It's not only that, Marilyn."

[You mean, you could just want a child?!]

Yeah, but I became convinced that people weren't clear enough about their deeper motivations.

In making these connections for herself, Marilyn was aware that her early parenting role had, in effect, overdeveloped her parental functions and had also caused other aspects of her self to remain in deep storage. It was from this deep storage that she was slowly emerging. For Marilyn, her maternal desire has had to do with the desire to bring parts of herself into real existence, rather than with having a "real" child to raise.

Marilyn's choice to remain child-free coincided with the pregnancy of her last close friend who was not already a mother. With other friend's motherhood had come a "loss of time and energy" devoted to the friendship, although the "quality" of the friendship had remained. When this last friend became pregnant Marilyn made a different kind of decision and chose to involve herself with this friend's pregnancy and the baby when he or she arrived. This is one kind of involvement that a woman with positive maternal feelings may embark on as it becomes clearer that she will not ever be a mother herself. In describing this parallel process, Marilyn says:

As I've gotten more comfortable with my decision I am more comfortable with her decision being different from mine. . . .

Gradually I'm feeling OK about being differentiated in general from other people. In a way <u>this</u> is my baby—my ability to be differentiating myself from other people. This is the form [my baby] has taken—that of my own psychological development.

Marilyn's private practice as a psychotherapist to adults and children is a strong feature of her present identity—one that makes full use of her "caretaking" functions from childhood and that "fulfills a mission of achievement." Her experience reflects a common theme among women in all three pathways. A creative activity, work or otherwise, is noted as carrying an important aspect of a woman's personal identity. Although her work no doubt carries a part of her creative self, Marilyn emphasizes that it is her art work that is much closer to her core self. A follow-up interview with Marilyn revealed that her art work has progressed from pastel sketches to more elaborate paintings and raku pottery. Of this she says:

The art part is closer to the creative as opposed to the work part, although I believe work can also be creative. But I believe in terms of my history that work has been a "you must produce," or caretaking, and I see the art just springing from inside me.

In reflecting on the factors of the past 25 years most influential to the shaping of her present identity, Marilyn noted several things frequently mentioned by the transformative women. The summer of 1968 (San Francisco's "Summer of Love") was when "the whole world shifted" for her. It "became a jumping-off point" from which she took "a different path in life." "Becoming a professional and being in a relationship with a man who is egalitarian" were mentioned in the same breath, focusing attention on the importance of the combined features of work and relationship for the lives of transformative women.

In comparing the first and second halves of her life, Marilyn describes the interlocking themes of midlife that face all adult women, mothers or not, as they establish a sense of personal identity beyond the role of "caretaker of others":

The first half of my life has been outer directed. In terms of image, in a way I do think of myself as Mother Marilyn, or already having been a mother in a lot of ways. And being extroverted and attentive to other's needs before my own, and that kind of thing. And also, along with that, the whole thing of becoming successful, achieving more and more goals. . . . I've been going through a midlife crisis. I feel so much more vulnerable, and I think that this is part of what it is going to be like for the rest of my life. I think, actually, I've been vulnerable all along, but I didn't know it. And that I've lived the first half of my life as though I'm not vulnerable, and as though I can just keep giving and doing and achieving.

[As if it's endless?]

Yeah, and I can't. I've got limits, and it's becoming increasingly clear to me. And I think the second half of my life, I'm not sure what form it's going to take, but I think it is going to be more inner directed. . . developing my own individuality rather than compulsively caretaking others. . . . An image I get of myself sometimes is just standing at a kitchen sink (in a cabin in the woods) looking out a window, in a flannel shirt and a pair of jeans. Not being anybody's therapist or mother. And I fantasize how wonderful it would be to be up there and have a studio to paint in, having a half a dozen clients. I'm feeling so much less achievement oriented. It has just collapsed, that whole thing has collapsed. . . it feels really odd to not be striving to become something else, to prove to myself or to the world that I'm "good enough." . . . It's really new for me to really be accepting that being myself, trying to be a decent therapist, and my creative work is good enough.

Conclusion

Maternal desire has a different value and meaning in each of these two quite different roads to child-free lives and adult female identities. Judith's and Marilyn's lives show us that positive as well as negative family histories may contribute to the making of a child-free life. For Marilyn, the need to not have a child for fear of being somehow unable to meet the demands of motherhood was balanced by a wish to be able to live up to the "image" that her own mother failed to personify. Like many child-free women from dysfunctional families, Marilyn said, "I wanted to heal the child within me" before having a child of her own. She wished to feel assured that she would not replicate her own dysfunctional family experience. Judith, on the other hand, carried no such worries from her family experience. She seemed to carry the legacy of "strong women" in her family forward in her own unique way. Each woman, in her own way, came say "I could have become a mother, but I really wanted to be and do something else." This capacity to hold onto a nonmaternal desire is the "masculine" energy often associated with the child-free woman. The transformative woman asks why this energy must be seen as masculine. Why can't it be the reclaiming of hitherto unrecognized aspects of feminine energy?

Despite their differing participation in the sociological movements of the 1960s and early 1970s, the period had an impact on them both. For each the cultural climate provided the ethos of breaking old cultural and gender forms. Both were supported in their personal explorations of new values and new ideas, ultimately leading both to choose a child-free life.

Paramount for both women was the need to make a connection with an essential aspect of themselves and expressing this essence in ways that precluded motherhood. Readers may find themselves reacting to their journeys with some discomfort. That there may be something disquieting in reading about a woman whose chosen path includes a choice not to be a mother indicates the degree to which gender identity and personal identity have been confused in the understanding of women; fewer such feelings generally arise upon reading of men whose chosen life paths exclude fatherhood.

The "traditional," the "transitional," and the "transformative" woman each provide a focus for one of three interwoven processes in which the woman who is not a mother must involve herself to secure a positive experience of adult identity. The traditional woman highlights the process of mourning the loss of a potential identity and/or relationship. The transitional woman embodies the struggle to become aware of the interplay between conscious and unconscious aspects of identity. The transformative woman illustrates the commitment of individual effort that this awareness requires in order to pursue a life of one's own.

The transformative woman clearly challenges the view that

woman is always meant to be primarily, or only, a caretaker. By developing alternative forms of creative work as the main focus of their lives, women like Judith and Marilyn are giving birth to additional forms for female identity. Although society as constituted in the past has had little need of alternative ways of being for women, a future society based on humanity rather than gender will increasingly need diversity from both men and women.

For both these women, the deeper connection with the self evolved through meaningful relationships with others as much as it did through their own solitary efforts to be open to what was emerging from within. This means of accessing the creative space within oneself through intimate connection with others and permitting the self to be filled by what is there rather than designing a mission or plan represents a little-explored path of adult identity development, one that may be related to "feminine" characteristics seen in their most positive form. "Womb envy" may not be limited to a woman's reproductive capacity, but to this special way of developing an identity.

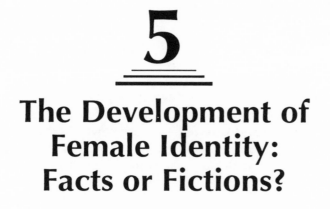

The Development of
Female Identity:
Facts or Fictions?

I continue to be amazed about how invested people are in
women being mothers. Most people tell me I would have been
a great mom and they think it's a shame because the world
needs mothers like me . . . I think it is threatening to be
childless. It's kind of like they are not able to keep you in "your
place."

In this chapter I will review how female identity has been
conceptualized from multiple perspectives and the way in which
these perspectives have influenced how "childless" women may
think of themselves. I will then have a basis to transform the
negative psychological portrait of the childless woman in psychology and psychoanalysis to offer a nonpathological model of her
development in Chapter 6. I begin with Sigmund Freud's views in
which he used maleness as the standard by which female identity
and "femininity" are defined. From there I move to the early
Freudian dissenters who countered with "femaleness" as its own
standard. The development of gender identity will then be placed
within the context of the scientific studies of the last half of the
century that appear to support Freud's dissenters. Continuing in
this direction I summarize the feminist rebuttal to Freud. Finally I
summarize female and male identity as they have been discussed by

the analyst Jacques Lacan and discuss how these ideas can help to make a positive niche in psychological theory for women who aren't mothers.

Sigmund Freud: The Primacy of Maleness

Freud believed girls and boys develop similarly prior to the oedipal stage. He conceived of sexual libido as being essentially "male" in character—active and directed outward toward others. In infancy and through early childhood, he thought the girl to be unaware of her vagina, but aware of her possession of a clitoris, which he viewed as an analog of the penis.[1] Since libido is active–aggressive, the girl child, in order to assume her heterosexual feminine role, must undergo a psychic transformation in the oedipal phase whereby the original active sex drive of infancy becomes passive. Several psychic maneuvers are necessary for the girl to achieve this transformation: she must shift her love from mother to father, renounce clitoral masturbation in preparation for acceptance of heterosexuality, and shift her sexual focus from clitoris to vagina. No such transformation is necessary for boys to adopt their heterosexual masculine roles.

Freud hypothesized that the dawning curiosity regarding sexual differences, and the realization that boys possess something (the penis) that girls do not, causes girls to be disappointed with their lack. Consequently they direct anger at the mother for not providing the penis (as well as anger because mother does not have one) or the girls think that they had one but that it was taken away (castration). This awareness, according to Freud, prompts the girl to seek substitutes for the penis, in order to resolve her sense of missing something. The search for a substitute penis is the essence of the girl's oedipal crisis. Freud saw three ways in which this crisis could be resolved. She can accept passive sexuality and resign herself to her feminine sex role, seeking from her father a baby as a replacement for the missing penis. She can renounce sexuality altogether. In the third possibility, the girl's psychic growth becomes fixed at the level of a "masculinity complex"; penis envy is never resolved. Thus the idea of penis envy becomes Freud's explanation for the girl's turning to her father as her primary love object; her wish for a child is a symbolic substitute for that which she can never have.[2] Though not expressed in Freud's formulations, an extension of his logic would equate voluntary childlessness with unresolved penis envy, and continuation of a "masculinity complex." A woman like Judith (Chapter 4) who pursued physics and then her own creative impulse, thereby foregoing family, would surely be viewed in this light.

A related aspect of Freud's understanding of female identity development was elaborated by Helena Deutsch, who considered masochism to be an essential expression of feminine nature.[3] Masochism results from the girl relinquishing an active–aggressive stance as she shifts her sexual focus from the clitoris (symbolic of activity) to the vagina (symbolic of passivity). A girl's aggression is thus turned inward towards herself rather than being able to be directed outwards. Added to this inwardly directed aggression is a wish to be sexually penetrated by the father as a masochistic repetition of what she perceives as her earlier castration and loss of her own penis. Female sexual relations with men in adulthood then become unconsciously linked with passivity and humiliation, and the pain–pleasure of childbirth are reminders of the girl's original castration.[4]

Freud and those theorists who elaborated his view of development used maleness as the benchmark for female identity. In these explanations there is no sense of male and female as two different but equal forms, but a sense of one developmental line—male development, with female development seen as based on a biological "lack." In classical psychoanalytic theory then, female identity is a secondary formation, not a primary one, and is based on an inherent, biologically based, insufficiency—the lack of a penis. Freud's comment that "anatomy is destiny" appears to ground his theory on a biological basis. Aspects of his theory, however, highlight the effect of symbolic meanings attached to the biological body. For example, a woman's wish for a child is viewed not as a uniquely female drive, grounded in female biology, but as a displaced wish for the missing male penis. Many women, in particular "traditional" women like Martina or Diane (Chapter 2), would find this assertion preposterous.

The fact that Freud's ideas have been questioned almost from their inception is due in part to Freud's own ambiguities and conflicts regarding the direct impact of the physical body on gender identity development and the effect on the development of female and male identity of symbolic meanings grafted upon biological differences between the sexes.[5] This conflict has been addressed by Freud's colleagues in different ways.

Early Psychoanalytic Dissenters

Some of Freud's contemporaries challenged his explanation of female identity as "lacking," instead suggesting original feminine strivings in girls' development.[6] Melanie Klein, Karen Horney, and Ernest Jones all countered Freud's notion that there was no vaginal awareness in infancy.[7] They suggested that the vagina, as an opening in the body, may be perceived as a continual threat to the body's integrity. Thus early awareness of the vagina may indeed be repressed, but repression differs from lack of recognition altogether.

These writers also reported differences in girls' and boys' behavior prior to the genital period, when gender identity is supposedly constituted. Their arguments support a view of gender identity as having developmental antecedents other than the resolution of the oedipal stage, and contradict the view of female identity as a secondary process resulting from a psychic transformation of a biological deficit. Diane (Chapter 2), whose earliest memories are of caring for her dolls like they were her own babies. comes to mind here. Her sense of herself as a mother and her wish for a child cannot be convincingly squeezed into the formulation of baby as a penis substitute.

Karen Horney offered an alternative viewpoint on penis envy and the role of envy in general based on sexual difference. From her perspective, "primary penis envy" in girls is related to young children's normal overevaluation of the urinary function, their exhibitionistic wishes for attention, and their suppressed masturbation desires that become aroused when seeing how boys can handle themselves during urination. Freud's concept of penis envy is seen by Horney as a transitory phase of female development during which the girl sees the obvious and real differences in the status of women versus men in society. Horney called this "secondary penis envy." Both Freud and Horney define the "masculinity complex" as a girl's rejection of the limited, socially prescribed role for women, achieved by keeping her primary identification with her father,[8] but Horney's description has a stronger sociocultural cast than Freud's intrapsychic focus. Horney also postulated a masculine version of penis envy, theorizing that boys and men envy women's reproductive capacity. Because boys do not have the physical capacity to bring forth a child from their bodies, Horney suggested that it is male envy of the womb that leads men to compensate for their lack by striving to get and maintain control over women and women's bodies. This patriarchal agenda leads some women, in an effort to maintain their own psychic and physical integrity, to forego the traditional feminine gender role either by choosing not to have children at all or maintaining an active masculine identification even if they do have children.

Horney's theory of identity development also reflects one gender's experience—but she focuses on the female experience. Her three personality organizations, resulting from failure to have basic security needs met in childhood, apply more directly to typically female rather than male experiences.[9] Horney noted that female children are subject to twin dangers within the nuclear family. Girls are subject to being sexualized and objectified by men and devalued by women. Though these dangers invariably evoke fear and anger in the girl, these feelings must be repressed for the sake of survival. In their place she develops an idealized female self that draws on cultural stereotypes regarding female identity and femininity. The development of an idealized and culturally determined sense of the female self leaves adult women constantly vulnerable to fears regarding their femininity, and can result in a "compulsive femininity" in an effort to secure emotional safety from assaults from father and brothers, and later from other boys and men.[10] Horney notes that the wish for a child can be either a real feminine drive or an attempt to fulfill the ideal of femininity. This kind of attempt can be seen in women whose drive to have a child takes on the compulsive quality of a goal to be met rather than a desired relationship. Horney's ideas suggest that there is a primary femininity in girls; she also stresses intrapsychic conflict in female identity development, but her work begins to address the strong social (patriarchal) forces at work in shaping female identity in a certain direction. The "transitional" woman's experience of conflict as expressed by Karen (Chapter 3), who both wanted a child and creative work, illustrates how these twin desires in a woman can be difficult to fulfill in a patriarchal society.

A Biosocial Frame for Gender Identity

Despite acknowledging some biological underpinnings, early analytic writers stressed the primacy of intrapsychic conflict for identity development, including gender identity. Freud took male development to be representative of human development, whereas Horney held female development to be more representative. In the 40 years since those writings, scientific findings have confirmed the views of Freud's dissenters more often than those of Freud himself. Subsequent scientific studies have supported the idea of young girls' awareness of their vaginas[11] and refuted the view of vaginal orgasm as "mature" and more representative of healthy adult female sexual experience.[12]

Freud described the girl as starting like a "little man," with masculine expressions of libido; prenatal studies reveal that all human embryos begin as "female," with transformation to male-ness dependent on the production of androgens to initiate the process.[13] Thus it may be more accurate to speak of the primacy of femininity in human development. Observational studies of young children have also shown that little girls express a greater interest in babies than do boys at ages prior to the oedipal period (the period at which, according to Freud's psychosexual theory, the wish for a child occurs in an effort to obtain a substitute penis).[14] This suggests there may be a preoedipal, hormonally based "feminine drive" that is missing in boys. Indeed, some of the women interviewed said that as long as they could remember they had always wanted a child.

The idea that feminine interest in babies and motherhood is biologically based has been supported in part by the research of Money and Ehrhardt on genetic sex disorders.[15] Children born with external female genitalia who are chromosomally and hormonally male may be raised as girls and form stable female gender identities, but may express little or no desire to have a child. This is also often true of female children who have been prenatally exposed to externally derived androgens, most often in an attempt to prevent miscarriage. These latter children develop stable female gender identities, but their gender role behavior is often more androgynous in nature—more tomboyish. This research brings to mind those women who told me that they had never enjoyed playing with dolls as a child and did not experience a strong drive to have a child.

Although the research on genetic sex disorders partially supports a biological base for the female desire for children, it also demonstrates the complex interplay of biological and psychological influences upon gender identity and gender role development. In the presence of a genetic sex disorder, either sex can be successfully assigned to a child, so long as this occurs prior to 18 months of age, when a core sense of gender identity becomes established. Cases of biological gender ambiguity can be resolved through medical intervention, but the treatment by parents of their child as a "girl" or a "boy" is a prime determinant for healthy gender development. It should be noted that both conscious and unconscious aspects of the parents' treatment of the child shape her or his gender identity and gender role. Diane's resolution of her infertility involved both conscious and unconscious identifications with her mother and her father. These enabled her to establish an alternative adult identity as a nurse and teacher, while at the same time fulfilling by displacement some of her strong maternal needs.

Robert Stoller's research on core gender identity has shown that gender identity, although still fluid, develops well before the oedipal period.[16] Daniel Stern's infant research also indirectly supports Stoller's work. Infants have a greater awareness of gender differences than has been assumed by psychoanalytic theorists; they also have a greater capacity for experiencing separateness and being-in-relationship.[17] Although gender identity is not specifically addressed, Stern's explorations have, in effect, deepened the biological roots and extended the psychological floor of identity development to the preoedipal years, years neglected by Freud.

This extension has implications for both female and male development. Irene Fast's gender differentiation theory shows that children in the preoedipal period are "overinclusive" in their ideas as to what female and male gender and gender role may include.[18] A little boy may still hold the notion that he, too, may have a baby, like his mother. In the oedipal period there is a sense of loss and a renunciation of the opposite sex, as gender identity consolidates. In this period, however, Fast notes that though capacities associated with the opposite sex may be renounced, other identifications may continue. Thus, a little girl may give up her idea that her penis will grow, but still retain a positive sense of assertion and aggression in her identity.

Together with the concept that gender identity development begins in the preoedipal period has come an examination of the maternal role in the development of a female identity. Current infant research stresses the importance of nonverbal, affective communication between mother and infant and its role in the infant's development of a secure and stable self. The mother's conscious and unconscious attitudes toward her daughter are perceived by some contemporary theorists as having a greater influence on positive female identity and role development than do the specific effects of the daughter's discovery of sexual difference in terms of her own and her mother's missing penis. The effect of these attitudes in developing an atypical female identity is revealed by Judith, who said that her mother's and grandmother's strength and positive attitude developed in her the sense that women could do so many things that she had always considered herself "automatically a feminist." From another vantage point some transitional women could be seen to carry their mothers' unacknowledged or unconscious wishes for more involvement in the world outside of the family.

Feminist Challenges

The Primacy of Mother: The Shift from Oedipal to Preoedipal

The British school of object-relations theory that emerged from the work of Melanie Klein, W. R. D. Fairbairn, and D. W. Winnicott has been particularly influential among American theorists taking up the banner of Freud's early dissenters. In highlighting the fact that it is a woman who is the primary caretaker for both female and male children, and that this impacts identity formation differently for females and males, object-relations theory has emphasized the importance of the preoedipal period and the crucial themes of relatedness and healthy interdependency for female and male identity development. British object-relations theory did not address gender directly, but Nancy Chodorow's analysis of the life-shaping and long-lasting differential influence of mother as woman upon both female and male identity has brought this aspect to light.[19]

Although object-relations theory is descriptive of both male and female identity development, feminists have used it in especially meaningful ways to understand how female identity is woven within interpersonal relationships. According to Chodorow, the girl's difficulty in life will be the formation and maintenance of an identity separate from her mother. This difficulty arises from the mother's (presumed) greater identification with her female baby than with her male baby, based on their shared gender. Although this greater identification may complicate the process of separation–individuation for the daughter, more fluid ego boundaries between daughter and mother can also enhance the development in the daughter of a greater capacity for empathic relatedness in her life. Unlike the male, who must reject his early identification with mother and shift his identification to father, the daughter's identity evolves through a path of continual relatedness; she will never have to completely relinquish her earliest maternal identification. Chodorow concludes that "feminine personality comes to define itself in relation and connection to other people more than the masculine personality. For boys and men, individuation and dependency issues become tied up with their sense of masculinity. . . . For girls, issues of femininity, or feminine identity, are not problematic in the same way" (Chodorow, 1978, pp. 45–46).

Within Chodorow's analysis of female identity development, "the reproduction of mothering" continues with women as primary caretakers because women yearn for the intimate bond of infancy with their mothers that then becomes replicated by having their own child. The implicit assumption here is that all female children will grow up to become mothers. The yearning for the bond of infancy is not missing in all women who are not mothers, it is, rather, worked out in a different arena. I believe that it is a common assumption that female childlessness is a result of pathological mothering. This assumption neglects the idea that for the women who do become mothers, not only is the lost *positive* infantile connection with their mothers reestablished but also the *negative*. This negative tie must be dealt with consciously to avoid repeating the same difficulties and woundings. In fact Chodorow sets her relational analysis within the patriarchal context and calls for more "coparenting" in families as a means to alter mothers' overinvolvement (and father's underinvolvement) in childrearing.

Drawing on biological differences and the object-relations idea of development as it occurs within a relational matrix, Jean Baker Miller and her colleagues at the Stone Center offer yet another feminist critique of the traditional oedipal story of female identity.[20] In this theory females are assumed to be of a different nature than males (similar to Horney's work). Feminine qualities of empathy, relatedness, and nurturance are revalorized, and the social and political context of patriarchy that has disavowed the feminine is stressed. Female identity is conceptualized as a "self-in-relation-ship" and is seen as developing from the matrix of the early preoedipal mother–daughter relationship. Miller and her colleagues propose the mother–daughter dyad as an alternative model of identity, in contrast to a male-biased model of identity that stresses autonomy and separateness. Martina's (Chapter 2) relationship with her mother in its capacity for mutuality and acceptance of difference clearly played an important role in Martina's integrating the meaning of infertility. Mutuality in relationship as seen in the mother–daughter pair is thus offered by the Stone Center as a model of how an "ethics of care" can be elaborated at both an individual and cultural level.[21]

Feminist research illuminates the difficulty of maintaining a positive female identity into adolescence and adulthood, a difficulty accentuated if a woman does not become a mother. This difficulty is based in part on the classical view of feminine development as a departure from the masculine norm. One of Freud's conclusions regarding the differing female resolution of the Oedipus complex was that women develop a weaker superego than do men, based on his hypothesis that superego development is a result of fear of castration. Sociologist Carol Gilligan challenges this reading of the meaning of gender difference regarding the moral development of girls and boys.[22] Her study showed that girls' moral and ethical judgments are grounded in the relational context of the ethical question, whereas for boys, moral considerations reflect a reliance on abstract principles. The latter is generally considered to be a higher moral reasoning process. Gilligan's study places new value on traditionally feminine attributes and challenges the classical Freudian notion that women's superego functioning is inferior to that of men. Different forms of moral reasoning are seen to stem from different developmental processes, and the hierarchical evaluation of these processes is seen as a culturally based conclusion, rather than an intrinsic quality. Similarly, in *Women's Ways of Knowing*, Belenky, Clinch, Goldberg, and Tarule contrast the different ways women obtain knowledge with society's normative masculine model of acquiring and demonstrating knowledge.[23] Feminist research and the Stone Center's theoretical work provide a sociopolitical context for understanding the devaluation of women and draw positive portraits of the feminine as something essentially different from the masculine self, offering a different but equal model of sexual difference.

Supporting the sociocultural antecedents of Horney's view of the twin dangers for girls of sexualization and evaluation, recent research by Gilligan reveals how an essentially positive sense of identity in young girls becomes negatively distorted and eroded in adolescence by the social/sex role demands to assume the role of a "desirable female." The self-esteem and academic performance of an adolescent girl appear to decrease in direct proportion to the degree to which she takes on the traditional cultural stereotype of "woman" as a part of her own identity.[24] In *The Girl Within*, Emily Hancock recounts the process by which adult women psychically return to their childhood selves to reconnect with their lost, positive female selves.[25]

The feminist interpersonal–social learning perspective can appear to overemphasize and overidealize the mother–daughter bond to such a degree that it is unimaginable why or how a woman would ever choose not to become a mother herself, or how she could ever develop a positive sense of identity if childbearing is denied her for physical reasons. The typical mother–daughter relationship that always includes some hate as well as love, and how this influences the women who do become mothers, is missing. In attempting to redress the Freudian emphasis on female development as a departure from a masculine norm and the Freudian neglect of the effect of early, preoedipal life on gender development, the Stone Center model however is emphasizing female development as its own, equally valid, development track and emphasizes particular aspects of early mother–daughter relationships.

The Stone Center approach has not, up to this point, explicitly addressed female identity apart from motherhood. Father is also missing in the Stone Center's approach to female identity as he is in object-relational theory (just as mother and femaleness is missing in early Freudian accounts of female identity). The Stone Center's relational model of female identity differs from object-relations theory in that the influence of the unconscious on human identity is little explored. Unconscious processes, from this point of view, seem to be limited to those aspects of one's self that must be disavowed in order to preserve a connection with another. From this perspective, the idea of a woman growing up with motherhood not being central to her identity may seem even more unusual, if not pathological, because of the absence of a more fully developed idea of the unconscious and the emphasis on defining a specifically female course of development as separate but equal to that of males.

In summary, psychological theories view either maleness (oedipal father) or femaleness (preoedipal mother) as the central organizer of female identity, with biology and culture as contextualizing influences. Yet regardless of whether maleness or femaleness is seen as the primary influence, maternity is still considered the equivalent of adult female development. There is no normative female identity for the woman who is not a mother.

Female Identity in Flux: The Problem of Symbolic Representation and Female Subjectivity

In order to begin to make a normative place for a different adult female identity I would like to return to an original Freudian conflict. This conflict concerns whether Freud thought the physical body was primary in determining identity development (i.e., anatomy is destiny) or whether the unique symbolic capacity of human beings, epitomized in language, was the predominant effect in shaping identity development. Jacques Lacan, also a controversial analyst, revisioned Freud in terms of the symbolic. Elements important for a new view of female identity are Lacan's shift of the emphasis of the oedipal crisis from Freud's biologically based understanding of identity to a theory of human subjectivity in terms of how language structures identity, and his reformulation of the role of the father.[26]

Lacan's revision of the oedipal crisis clearly falls on the symbolic side of Freud's conflict regarding the role of the body in identity development. The function of the father, as Lacan saw it, was to provide the needed "third term," inaugurating the infant's process of separation–individuation from the psychic orbit of the mother; father facilitates the shift of the seemingly fused "unit" of mother–infant to two separate beings—mother *and* child. This heralds the beginning of the acquisition of a separate identity in the child and the development of the child's capacity for language, which are intricately connected. (It is important to note here that the oedipal drama may in fact involve the father's presence as the "third term," or may be carried "symbolically" in the mother herself, through her attitude toward the father and/or the social laws represented by the paternal name given to the child.) The oedipal prohibition is the interdiction preventing the mother from keeping her child within her own psychic boundaries (a broader prohibition than incest). Only through this psychic separation–individuation process can the child take her or his named identity within the family and society.

The acquisition of language is key in assuming a separate human identity. This capacity is, however, a double-edged sword; it is what makes us uniquely human and different in the animal kingdom, yet it alienates us from ourselves because language never adequately expresses our experiences. The separation and partial psychic loss of the infant–mother relationship through repression of infancy is experienced by every person as the price paid for becoming a fully functioning person ("subject," in Lacanian terms). This loss, common to us all, has significant implications for the societal meaning of femininity and masculinity.[27]

Theoretically, either parent could assume the role of this "third term," facilitating a child's psychic separation from the symbiotic orbit of the primary parent. In fact, women, as mothers, have historically been in the position of the primary parent who must be left. Partially as a result of this traditional parental arrangement, femaleness has become unconsciously connected to loss and the unspeakable because, as our separate sense of self solidifies, our infancy fades into unconsciousness. Father symbolizes the prohibition against a never-ending, seamless connection between mother and child that, if left uninterrupted, would leave the child in a state of psychosis; there would be no psychic differentiation from the body or psyche of the "(m)Other." Maleness often acquires a consciously positive value because father is associated with the authority and power that comes with the new self-awareness of a conscious identity separate from mother. These associations are then carried unconsciously by both women and men, and serve as the substrate of institutionalized sexism.[28]

The phallus unconsciously represents the paternal intervention into the mother–child relationship that permits the beginning of a conscious sense of one's self. Each individual organizes her or his identity in relation to this symbolic intervention of the father, because each person must fill in a named place (given to us before birth) within a society whose rules and expectations for human behavior preceded our birth. Female identity is clearly a "lack" in this revisionist Freudian view because no girl child can look to her own phallus, but the "lack" in Lacanian theory is a symbolic one and is specifically expressed in terms of a linguistic position. To hold a female position is to be identified with all within ourselves that is unconscious and/or cannot be consciously spoken; a male position is to be identified with a conscious identity and all that can be spoken. The fact that femaleness and maleness are *positions* in relation to language in identity and are not inherently *biological facts* is what is useful here.

Lacanian analysis is a description of patriarchy and how it is psychically maintained. It also contains within it the means for its undoing, because both women and men may take a feminine or masculine position in relation to their own identity or that of others. The meaning of the capacity to shift linguistic positions in relation to one's own identity is made particularly concrete and understandable when looking at the pathway of the transitional women (Chapter 2). These women spend periods of time in which the issue of motherhood for their identity is not consciously addressed. It is in the background because they are simply living in the stream of their lives. There are other periods when the question of motherhood is in bold relief for these women and everything in the stream of their lives is consciously framed by how motherhood contributes to the meaning and form of their adult female identities. June (Chapter 3) is an excellent example of this process in action.

An important question for women in general—how do women situate themselves symbolically in society in their own female terms? How do women, mothers or not, represent their experiences in everyday language when much of female experience in society is left unspoken.

Feminists have recently been dealing with the question of female identity per se within the context of language's central importance for human identity. In a typically European fashion, exalting "la différence," Luce Irigaray, a French analyst, agrees with Lacan that language has been co-opted by the masculine and by men, and says a "double syntax" is needed.[29] As Irigaray sees it, female experience cannot ever be fully expressed in our present-day masculine-biased language; women need to develop an alternative use or kind of language to represent female experience. Irigaray directly challenges the traditional dichotomy of maleness and femaleness, seeing it as a false and nonexistent dichotomy. In her view "Woman" is not really "Other," but only an "Other of the Same"; a male projection about woman and a place of residue where "He" is not (she is described only in terms relative to the masculine). Patriarchal society depends on a different Other, so to speak, existing; but in reality Woman as a real Other is not fully manifest—what is manifest is always disavowed. Patriarchal society requires that someone other than men exist to establish and maintain a heirarchy whereby maleness is designated superior and men retain power. Women, instead of being defined in truly different or "other" terms of their own however, are defined in terms of a negation—femaleness is whatever is not male. Femaleness not expressed in terms of negation is disavowed altogether and denied representation and or valuation in society (i.e., women's kind of interpersonal focus in their development). Because female experience and the female unconscious are not fully represented linguistically, and cannot be within our current masculine symbolic system of language, the task for women, as Irigaray sees it, is to create and produce "women's writing." Only through this writing can women claim their own destinies, desires, and full female subjectivity. This link is seen in the 42-year-old woman who said that when her desire to have a child stirred, so did the desire to write.

Of special relevance for the identity of childless women is Irigaray's discussion of the feminine as equivalent to melancholia because there is no representation of the loss between mother and daughter as the daughter passes through the oedipal complex—in effect there is no female lineage. A daughter who is given the surname of her mother or grandmother cannot be represented as "Mary Stewart II," because the family name of the mother is generally not symbolized. Female lineage is not maintained symbolically as it is for males; when the daughter has children of her own she simply takes the place of her mother with no symbolic representation in the language of society of her differentiation from her mother (e.g., there is no Mary III). Thus the daughter's identity appears, according to Irigaray, as one continuous thread with her mother's. (Naomi Lowinsky's *The Mother Line* is a study of a female lineage of this sort.) The significant number of daughters not taking their mothers' places suggests a female lineage is beginning; these daughters are making a break, a social discontinuity in the continuous thread of adult female identity as mothers. By dedicating one of her books to her mother, Judith (Chapter 4) was making a link between two very different female lives of daughter and mother.

Julia Kristeva, another French analyst, also addresses the problem of representing female experience in language but from a somewhat different perspective. She describes the preoedipal maternal period as a semiotic (sign) mode of representation and the oedipal paternal period as one of symbolic (linguistic) representation. Yet Kristeva also espouses a classically Freudian (and Winnicottian) idea in her suggestion that the bisexual nature of human beings means that all aspects of signification or representation are possible (both in semiotic and symbolic realms) and that identity exists only in the dialectic between the symbolic and semiotic layers of individual experience.[30] In other words, the essence of human identity is always somewhere between what is unspeakable and spoken—somewhere between what is female and male.

Kristeva has some very interesting ideas regarding motherhood and what motherhood does or does not offer in terms of representing female subjectivity. For the childless woman, her ideas concerning gender as a discontinuous category are more salient. Her concept of the "subject in process" describes a model of identity as "always becoming" due to the continual dialectic of the semiotic and symbolic. This focus upon taking a conscious stance regarding one's own conscious and unconscious (as the "Other" within) in an active dialectic suggest a model of how a childless woman may approach her female identity and her own, or culturally attributed, experience of her "missing or absent child." (I will be describing this process for of her "missing or absent child." (I will be describing this process for each of the traditional, transitional, and transformative women in Chapter 6.)

With a more typically American emphasis on the inherent equality of the sexes, theorist Jane Gallop takes a different approach to the problem of registering feminine experience in language. She takes the position that all human beings are "subject" to the same laws of language in becoming a human being, but sight (by which one discerns the presence or absence of a penis) has become especially privileged. The task of women currently is to elaborate other senses and signs of sexual difference heretofore devalued and linguistically impoverished (such as the olfactory sense) because of being associated with the feminine as the unspeakable, or devalued and disallowed[31] (à la Irigaray). Consider how few words there are to elaborate the olfactory and tactile senses—both of which are associated more with femaleness—compared to those for the visual and auditory senses. How do we begin to think and speak from and through the female body? is the question Gallop asks. (Significantly, she does not ask how we speak from the maternal body.)

Another Lacanian notion of particular importance for female identity and especially childless women is that of the "third term." The "third term" and its effects for human identity and subjectivity have been taken up in a recent object-relational analyses of female development by Jessica Benjamin. Benjamin focuses on the role of the preoedipal father for the girl child—the figure usually missing in object-relational theory.[32] In an oblique Lacanian reference, Benjamin says that, for girls, there is no real "third" to introduce her into a full subjectivity of her own. Girls have no relationship in which mutuality and recognition of a separate identity are possible in the way they are for boys, who receive recognition of their separate and independent identities within a male gender identity, represented by their fathers. (This view can be seen to represent the "flip side" of Chodorow's view that males have a more difficult time consolidating gender identity due to the need to separate by gender from the original symbiotic partner. Of course many traditional fathers may give their son "recognition" but still not be available often enough to help the boy fill out the meaning of "maleness.")

Whereas both the girl and the boy will look to the father as the third, that someone to support individuation and separation from though this is certainly not true for all sons). This recognition helps to consolidate the boy's personal independence within a male gender identity.

To remain strongly identified with mother in a patriarchal culture gives a girl a secure sense of gender identity, but often leaves her with an impaired sense of personal independence and of her ability to act on her own desires, particularly when mother is perceived as somehow "less" independent and capable than father. In the traditional family grouping the girl often has no independent figure available to assist in her own consolidation of a sense of individual "agency" within a female gender identity. Among the traditional women especially and also some of the transitional women, there was a sense that they had difficulty imagining their lives without motherhood, in part because they had no sense of their mothers' competency and confidence beyond the confines of the maternal role.

Benjamin describes a conflicted gender identity as one of the difficulties and dangers that can ensue when a girl tries to use her father as a representative of the outside world and a model of personal independence and agency. This state of affairs is reflected in the lives of some transitional women like Karen (Chapter 3) who tried to deny her own independent strivings because she saw them as masculine.

Benjamin raises the serious question of how women can be expected to become "desiring subjects" (rather than merely the objects of male desire) when a viable "third" is missing to facilitate the recognition and integration of personal agency within a stable female gender identity. As Benjamin sees it, the absence of this "third" can lead the girl to overidealize maleness as representing a sense of agency, and she may then tend to submit to masochistic relationships with men in an attempt to gain recognition of her own sense of agency through a psychic merger with them. (By psychically merging with the sadist [master], the masochist [slave] briefly experiences an empowered identity of being a master.)

Summary and Conclusion

Female identity and femininity have been and remain the Bermuda Triangle of psychoanalytic theory. It is fair to say that all psychological theories suggest, in one way or another, that a "woman's reproductive capacity shapes her mental life."[33] Yet a woman's capacity to give birth need not be seen only in the context of her capacity to produce biological children. Because there is no positive representation of the feminine apart from maternity, our theories concretize female destiny rather than seeing a woman's reproductive capacity as an organic basis for developing many feminine symbols or metaphors. This concretization creates a problem in the telling of the story of "the individual" from a truly female perspective, unless we take recourse to fixed notions of femaleness as equated to maternity.

An important intersection in the psychoanalytic theories of female development that directly concerns the female identity of the women who are not mothers is this question of the "third." Language is the "third term" in adult identity that opens a reflective space between one's self and one's immediate experience. Given that there is a virtual absence of female experience in language other than by reference to the masculine, there is little possibility of expressing exclusively female experience. It is in this sense that "woman" is seen by some to not yet exist. Irigaray argues that femaleness is not "one" (like the phallus) but multiple, diffuse in pleasure, and requires linguistic representation on its own terms, and not in terms related to male experience. Jane Gallop would not suggest a separate syntax like Irigaray but she sees the need for women to claim and express their experiences in language since she sees language as neutral (although she does not deny the effects of a present masculine bias) and synonymous with the human condition.

Many women, according to Jessica Benjamin, are lacking a full subjectivity of their own to express because of the absence of a viable "third" in the family that could facilitate a daughter's efforts to attain her own subjectivity and a sense of herself as equal but different from maleness. In those families where mother is not an independent person, daughters must search for a "third term" by which a fuller subjectivity may be developed. This might be accomplished by looking within and taking an active position in their own conscious–unconscious dialectic (as Kristeva discusses), in relationship to females outside the family, or in some combination of internal and external exploration.

It is the first time in history that women have an array of reproductive choices before them, including the choice not to be a mother. These choices make more room for an expanding female identity. Some of the new possibilities for female identity are being explored by women who have assumed neither the role nor identity of mother. Whether we think of these women as childless or child-free women, women who are able to develop satisfactory "atypical" female identities represent, to date, an unconscious element in our theories of gender development. The discovery of the unconscious itself by Freud as the absent but present place in each personality expanded our understanding of the meaning and complexity of the human psyche. So, too, women who aren't mothers, absent in psychological theory but always present in reality, lead us to expand our interpretations of female subjectivity and challenge our simplistic notions of gender and gender roles. Today these women are actively pushing against the boundaries of psychological theory by living at the margin of sexual difference, gender, and gender roles as we have known them. The following chapter presents a way in which women who are not mothers may begin to be included in psychological theory.

6

Weaving an
Alternative Understanding

With a wall around
A clay bowl is molded;
But the use of the bowl
Will depend on the part
Of the bowl that is void.
　　　—Tao Te Ching

That "women" is impossible and indeterminate is no cause for
lament.
　　　　　　　　　—Denise Riley

The lives of the 100 women I interviewed indicate it is necessary to
expand the "childless" woman's place in theory beyond the
parameters of deviance. The pathological view of these women in
psychological theory has for too long both influenced the way these
women are represented by others in society and limited the way
these women may think of themselves. Aspects of psychoanalytic
theory, however, can offer a perspective from which one might
begin to understand the woman who is not mother. Object-
relational and Lacanian theory each provide valuable ideas that the
other excludes; together they present another view on a childless
woman's identity development, one that considers this developmental path as a variation upon female identity development rather
than as an abnormal outcome.

These two threads of contemporary psychoanalysis emphasize different figures in the unfolding tapestry of identity development. Each uses as background what the other theorist regards as the primary figure. In object-relational theory, mother is the central organizing figure of identity; in Lacanian theory, it is the father. Yet both theories use concepts related to absence—"lack" (Lacan) or "potential space" (object-relations) with regard to personal identity. This is particularly important in understanding the childless woman, who is often perceived by society as a woman of absence.

Object-Relations Theory

Feminists drawing upon object-relations theory have perhaps tended to link "relatedness" and female identity too closely to motherhood per se. There is the tacit implication that women's capacity for empathic relatedness is necessarily developmentally fulfilled in motherhood.[1] This trend has had the effect of reinforcing the usual gender dichotomy by associating women with "related-ness" and men with "autonomy." Moreover, it splits off women who are not mothers into a theoretical cul-de-sac.

Based on the stereotype that the childless woman is the result of inadequate mothering, object-relations theory might explain the phenomenon of childlessness by postulating that a woman's pregnancy would trigger in her inner world a feeling of merger with the representation of the "bad mother" inside her; she will actively avoid motherhood in order not to contaminate her own separate positive female identity.[2] This theory supports the idea that some women eschew motherhood for fear of repeating a dysfunctional model of parenting.

An alternate view suggests that pregnancy activates in a woman an internalized relationship (object-relation) between a "good enough" mother and a poor or absent father; to bear a child would be to place herself (and her child) in such psychic jeopardy that she is unwilling to proceed with the pregnancy. In this view, motherhood is to be avoided not because of identification with a "bad mother" but because of identification with a "good mother" in a "bad relationship."

Both of these views stem from negative parental situations. These internal representations do account for some women who don't become mothers—but not all. The life histories of the 100 women interviewed suggest that childlessness is not invariably the result of dysfunctional parenting. The lives of the women discussed in Chapters 2-4 show that highly functional parents can produce daughters who are able to forge atypical, but positive, adult female identities.

All mothers are women, but not all women are mothers. (Neither has it ever been true that all mothers are the same.) Whereas feminist interpretations of object relations have emphasized the relatedness aspect of female identity development, object-relations theory can also discuss women whose identities do not include motherhood, without recourse to theories of pathological development. This more normative explanation can be linked to the idea of bisexuality.[3] British analyst D. W. Winnicott has broadened the concept of bisexuality beyond its sexual meaning to include the idea that the possibilities of "being" (stereotypically feminine) and "doing" (stereotypically masculine) are both present at the beginning of life and only become dichotomized according to gender when the child reaches the oedipal age. (This position is also taken by Julia Kristeva in regards to symbolic representation.) At this time culturally determined linguistic meanings and values regarding "being" and "doing" become associated with sexual differences.[4]

Current infant research seems to indicate that the infant's capacity for both relatedness and selfness is far greater than previously hypothesized. At the age of 7 weeks an infant can initiate a degree of mutuality in relationships to others simply by controlling her or his gaze.[5] The infant research of Daniel Stern compellingly suggests that there exists from birth an everpresent "arc of tension" between the poles of separation and relatedness; a dynamic tension existing in the child at increasing levels of sophistication as maturation unfolds. This research also adds credence to Nancy Chodorow and Dorothy Dinnerstein's thesis that it is likely that the structure of parenting (e.g., the mother as primary caretaker rather than the father) with regard to parental models of relatedness or autonomy determines many of the differences in the subjective experiences of females and males seen in later childhood and adulthood. Although individual differences in innate endowment also contribute to differences, innate sexual differences may not have the degree of impact that have been attributed to them.

Differences in style among primary caretakers may also help explain variations in female development, including the decision for childlessness or motherhood. Women have always had different desires and competencies, but the women of the 20th century have had the most opportunity to pursue them. The generation of women who filled the shoes of men during World War II had these privileges rescinded at war's end, but the desires kindled by these nontraditional experiences remained. Not surprisingly the daughters of these women have found their own ways of expressing these desires. Choosing not to bear children is one of them.

Mothers also vary in their degree of maternal ambivalence and in their allegiances to cultural norms regarding what female attitudes and behaviors should be. They offer to their daughters many versions of what a woman can be. The degree to which any child will manifest the usual stereotypical sex role characteristics or socially sanctioned heterosexuality within a specific gender identity will partially emerge from the child's relationship with her particular mother. A mother can, to a greater or lesser degree, model and reinforce socialized meanings given to sexual difference.

Until recently object-relations theorists have most often written about the mother–infant bond in terms of the child as subject and the mother as object.[6] Less attention has been given to consideration of the mother as a "subject" with her own desires, and to facets of her identity other than her caretaking attributes.

The child's discovery of the mother's own personality and subjective experience is a significant part of separation–individuation. Through repeated separations from the mother, empathic failures on the part of the mother, and through the infant's real and imagined aggression, the mother is discovered as a person who provides, rather than just being a providing environment. Through these processes a psychic space opens up between mother and child that Winnicott calls the "transitional or potential space." The child, in her or his earliest creative gesture, tries to fill this space by endowing certain objects and (later) words with mother's soothing functions. This initial use of transitional space is a necessary step towards internalizing the maternal functions as part of the infant's own psychic structure. (It is also the genesis of the creative act.)

During this process, the infant also discovers that mother is indeed a human being, separate and capable of being emotionally and physically damaged.[7] The infant gradually takes in consciously and unconsciously the realization that mother has desires other than being a mother (to be with others, creative labor, sleep, etc.).

Little has been written about this side of mother (mother as subject), other than mother's desire for father or relationship.[8] The female child will take in nonmaternal features as she comes to know them, and in some cases will unconsciously identify with these aspects of mother and later unconsciously and consciously act on these identifications. These features of identification with mother are represented within the inner theater of her own mind as part of what it means to be female,[9] and are available to her as a source of her own female identification in future years. Diane (Chapter 2) was obviously strongly identified with the maternal aspects of her mother, but she was also able to draw upon her mother's desire to be engaged in the world of work outside the home. In her career in nursing, Diane was able to draw upon both maternal and nonmaternal features of her mother as grounding for her female identity.

A girl may develop a personality organized around related-ness—or what is thought of as traditionally female. She may or may not have children. Alternatively, if her mother presents herself as a less "traditional" female, the girl's personality may become organized more around the "autonomy" pole of identity. A woman who is more autonomous and does not bear children can be so as a result of positive modeling by mother, not necessarily because of severe maternal ambivalence or in reaction to poor mothering.

Depending on the features her mother unconsciously and consciously models or supports, a daughter may become a woman whose personality is drawn to motherhood or gravitates elsewhere. Or, if a daughter must face the fact that her desire to become a mother is not realizable, she may draw upon these other features of her identification with her own mother to stabilize her different female identity.

Object-relations theory focuses upon the preoedipal period of identity development; identification with other significant females besides mother may also occur in a girl's childhood and later adult life. Approximately one-third of the women interviewed had a significant attachment in their youth to a woman who was not a mother. These women presented a different model of female identity for identification and, in the inner theatre of the minds of these developing girls, represented a part of what it means to be a "woman." In essence these "other women" served as the "third term" in the sense used by Lacan, by serving as the third element needed for a symbiotic unit to become two separate entities. By indicating the reality that women can be other than mothers, these women created a "space" between the daughter and her mother's identity—a space in which alternative female identities might be imagined. A childless aunt in a number of these women's lives showed them that a woman could be "quite happy without children," could be very "lively and fun."

Preoedipal Father in Object-Relations Theory

A different situation exists in a preoedipal relationship (birth to about age 4) where mother has in fact not been sufficiently identified with or empathically attuned to her daughter. In these circumstances, the female infant may turn toward the father, not for help in individuating, which many analytical theorists have discussed, but for the missing maternal functions. In this altered situation, when the female baby turns to the father for missing maternal function, he (a male) becomes the recipient of the female baby's earliest identification, rather than mother (a female). This change in the usual sequence of events is obviously significant for her future female identity development.[10]

The female child who turns to father for maternal functions often experiences a kind of double jeopardy. She is not going to want to give up her primary identification with father when she reaches the oedipal period and learns of sexual differences; now there is even more reason to reject mother as a primary role model. Mother, who was lacking in maternal nurturance, is now also lacking any real social status or value. This child can be left with a conflicted gender identity—knowing she is female but somehow feeling more male inside. In this way she could be seen as a "daughter of the patriarchy" rather than being a woman-centered woman. Her conflicted identity may not result in childlessness, but if she remains childless, this may further undermine her female identity. She will not receive the social recognition of her femininity that could serve to balance an inner male identification. Several women I spoke with related their difficulty in working through what they perceived as an overidentification with their fathers, or maleness.

All women need to have and reinforce links of their female identities that are not tied to motherhood. But for childless women who have been very father identified this is especially important. Sometimes these will be added female features that are modeled and admired for the first time by women they know in adult life. (These features may have been present in their mothers but never actualized.) For example, Martina (Chapter 2) met several women in the course of her work at a social service agency who offered a model of woman other than the primary homemaker model of her family of origin. For some women these attributes will be ones unconsciously associated with a female figure or figures from the past that now become a conscious part of their adult identities.

In general, however, the positive contributions of the father–daughter relationship to female gender identity and personal identity, especially an atypical one, have not been stressed enough in psychoanalytic theory. Jessica Benjamin in *Bonds of Love* has suggested that the preoedipal father can recognize a girl's emerging independent identity when mother has an adequate sense of self. The women interviewed who grew up in this kind of family constellation seem to carry with them a sense of "automatically being a feminist," as did child-free Judith of Chapter 4. They seem to assume naturally the prerogatives of what has been seen as a masculine gender role as a part of their own repertoire of attitudes and behavior.

Benjamin's work also stresses the potentially problematic outcome in the oedipal years and later when the preoedipal father is used as a source of what she calls "identificatory love"—the object who can recognize a daughter's sense of agency when the mother does not have an adequate sense of self. In this study, however, there did seem to be fathers who were able to receive both the (preoedipal) "identificatory love" from their daughters *and* the love and desire of the oedipal years in such a way that the daughters' autonomy developed within a coherent female identity, despite mother's lack of presence as a person in her own right. When this was the case, these women in adulthood were then able to challenge the existing social structures that attempted to limit their lives. One woman was able to pursue going to medical school in the face of an admissions officer saying he would accept 50 men before he would accept a woman, because of the personal agency her father's recognition of her had nurtured.

Shame has always been a powerful social tool to keep woman in her place as a mother, at home; many women continue to feel something is wrong with them if they don't have or want to have children. For some of the women interviewed, father was a significant reason why they were able to assert their female identities with confidence and without shame to those who inquired about or challenged their differentness (childlessness). One 41-year-old woman who had actively chosen a life apart from motherhood related her choice in part to a positive relationship with her father. He supported her developing competencies as a young girl with the same quality of energy that he directed towards his son's developing abilities:

> I was closer to my dad [than to my mother]. He and I did a lot
> of stuff together. He is the one who encouraged me, discour
> aged me. He was essentially my role model; he gave me a sense
> of who I am and what the world was like, and who I was, or
> could be, in the world. . . . In this respect, I'd like to think that
> how I was brought up was very nonsexist.

An irony here is that the identity development of most of these women corroborates a common notion among many theorists that relatedness, or relationships with others, is a major organizer of identity for women. They most often do report that their sense of self unfolds within the context of their relationships. But, since all childless women must develop their lives without the centrality of mothering, separation and autonomy are necessarily also very significant themes in their identities. Those women who seem to have organized their senses of identity around the pole of autonomy (most often the child-free, like Judith and Marilyn in Chapter 4) often have a coexisting sense of self embedded within a larger field of relatedness, for example, spirituality, or global and humanitarian issues. Thus even at their most autonomous, women seem to remain in a web of connection.

Thus, from an object-relations viewpoint both positive and negative pathways to female identities that do not include motherhood are possible, depending upon the particular configuration of the significant relationships in early life. Object-relations theory is concerned with the preoedipal years although it offers a model of how significant relationships in later life can also shift and modulate our internal ideas about ourselves and others. Yet object-relations theory does not address the organizing function of the oedipal drama for female and male gender identities. For this the Lacanian revision of the oedipal stage becomes relevant.

Lacanian Theory: Oedipal

A Lacanian psychoanalytic perspective supplements object-relations theory in elaborating on the role of the father in identity development and understanding its implications for childless women.[11] This theory stresses the meaning of the child's transition, which father facilitates, from the nonspeaking state of early infancy (the term "infans" literally means nonspeaking) to becoming a speaking being, capable of symbolic activity through the use of language. Every individual identity, female or male, is "lacking," in a sense, because the early psychic loss of the mother is constituted structurally within our personality as the unconscious—always experienced by the individual as the Other in her or himself. It is during the oedipal phase that this earlier psychic loss of mother is negated and then symbolized in the form of one visible sign of sexual difference—the penis.

The reification of the phallus in language has major psychic effects for both girls and boys. The phallus has come to unconsciously represent not only the "difference" between the sexes, but also a sense of the "oneness" or "wholeness" of individual identity. Women, who "lack" a penis, are invariably perceived as "lacking," whereas men are overvalued because they possess one. This *visible* sign of sexual difference (though not the only one), the penis, has become secondarily elaborated and valued in our patriarchal culture, thereby contributing to the power differential between woman and men.[12] Childless woman are only a special subset of the entire female gender, whose challenge it is to write themselves into his-story so it can also be her-story. The Lacanian emphasis on the role of language in constructing human identity and the place of women at the unspeakable helps us also see that childless women will especially be equated with "lack" so long as there is virtually no elaboration in social discourse on a woman's identity apart from motherhood.[13] Including these women in our theories of female development is a beginning.

The relationships some of the women interviewed had with their fathers show us that men can assist women in their efforts to add her-story to history, particularly in a parental situation. When fathers are able to recognize their daughters' emerging separate identities and speak directly about the daughter's personal agency in terms of her own gender identity and her place in the world, a greater appreciation of the difference between gender role and biological femaleness or maleness can develop in the daughter. One 50-year-old woman said:

> There's always been a more complex quality in the relationship between my father and I than between my mother and I. For my father's era he gave me a lot of freedom as a female that I think a lot of men his age did not allow their daughters. He supported my inquisitiveness and questioning of everything.

Another 46-year-old woman said of her father, "I give my father a lot of credit for my sense of independence, my sense of self, and my sense of separateness in this world. Also, my sense of my own value."

For women who had this type of father, more psychic differentiation developed between gender identity and personal identity—an especially important differentiation for girls, since gender and personal identity are more often seen as identical (or at least highly related) in girls than in boys. Gender developed then as a salient category for identity, but a category neither fixed in meaning nor limited to particular roles she might assume in her life. (It is this kind of shift in parental role in the nuclear family that Nancy Chodorow and Dorothy Dinnerstein had in mind in the 1970s.)

All women are faced with the dilemma of how to exercise their personal authority in our patriarchal society. This problem is perhaps only accentuated for childless women. Motherhood at least provides some measure of legitimate social standing, whether conceptualized as a "penis substitute" or as the fulfillment of womanhood. The women who aren't mothers must try to find a means of establishing personal and social authority apart from this traditional path; to date, there has been no way to do this without being masculinized or marginalized by theory and society.

Postoedipal Development: Figure(s) and Ground for Adult Identity

It is practically impossible to think of the woman who is not a mother without thinking of something absent, lacking, or missing, so prominently is motherhood woven into the social construction of the adult female identity. How can we think of this in theoretical terms for female identity? Lacanian theory emphasizes the notion of lack in terms of the unconscious—a universal human condition. Because the penis, symbolizing wholeness, has resulted in masculine characteristics becoming associated with positive value and presence whereas female characteristics have become associated with negative value and absence, the empty womb of the childless woman can be seen as a symbol of even greater absence. The childless woman's lack is thus simply more obvious than that of other women in her pronatal culture.

By approaching the theme of intersubjectivity, a net can be woven between object-relational and Lacanian theory to redefine that aspect of "absence" that belongs uniquely to the childless woman and to explore how this relates to her particular identity. Object-relational and Lacanian theories attend to the meaning of separation and loss in identity development, but each emphasizes a different figure (mother and father, respectively) and views the other as secondary to that process. Depending on one's perspective of figure and ground, the outcome for the meaning of the self is also different. Each perspective offers something for the woman who is not a mother.

A redefinition of the "place of absence" offers the greatest potential for developing a new meaning–symbolization of this concept. Both of these psychoanalytic perspectives ("transitional space" or "lack") regard a place of absence as the locus of desire and/or creativity. Both discuss to how one becomes more fully present through encountering one's absence. Each conceives of absence within the individual psyche as the space made between the mother and child, although they differ in their description of how this space comes into existence. Both perspectives agree that without this necessary psychic loss there would be no room for symbolization and the development of the self-reflective person to occur.[14]

Lacanian theory emphasizes the alien and external role of language in making possible the development of a subjective self. Language is the "third term" in human identity that functions to make metaphorization possible. It is the term that comes between ourselves and our own experiences to make the necessary space for self-reflection. (For example, in anticipating a gourmet meal, there is not only the experience of smelling a gourmet meal cooking, but there is an internal verbal commentary about the appealing fragrances, an interpretation through words of the various reactions or associations to this olfactory sensation. In this example, language is the third term needed to make an objective olfactory sensation into a truly subjective experience.) In these terms, encountering one's absence in order to act creatively, and with aliveness, would involve looking with interest at one's spontaneous fantasies and dreams, the gaps in one's flow of conversation, the unintentional ("Freudian") slips of the tongue, and all the mistaken actions which reveal the self (subject in Lacanian terms) of the unconscious, which can then yield to interpretation and metaphorization.

In contrast, Winnicott views the absence, or transitional space if you will, from an interpersonal perspective, emphasizing the relational quality and describing creative activity from its origin in the relationship between self and other. For Winnicott, absence is conceptualized as the intermediate area of experience that includes both Me and Not-Me, fantasy and reality, because it arises out of the original relationship with the mother. Although Winnicott acknowl-edged the necessity of the third term for making subjectivity possible, he emphasizes the mother's role in opening this space.[15] This "potential or transitional space" between infant and mother will be filled with various internal objects and language created by the child that serve to partially bridge the original psychic separation from mother. This original use of this space, this place of absence, is repeated throughout our lives. In our adult moments of creative work or play, which may indeed occur while being alone, we are also experiencing a deeply felt connection with the first Other. This connection with the first Other may have a particular meaning for the childless woman, whose creative urge may come in part from the yearning to reestablish her primal connection with the (m)Other and to reconnect with the earliest sources of her feminine self.

To combine these two views of absence and relate them to the adult experience of the childless woman, we could say that when a woman shifts her attention from experiencing childlessness as a concrete fact to wondering about the meaning of her childlessness for her life, she is introducing that "third term" of language between herself and her childless experience, making a psychic space where interpretation and elaboration of her own particular childlessness become possible. Only when this psychic shift occurs is she able to redefine the concrete absence as a "potential space" that she may enter and with which she may begin to create metaphors for her life as a part of consolidating a different female identity. One 46-year-old divorcee asserted her autonomous development by changing careers, and also filled the potential space (the "absence" of motherhood) by teaching dance—an activity that seemed to meld both her creative and generative needs.

The path to a satisfactory adult female identity for the woman who is not a mother must include encountering her own lack (as Lacanians would say), that of not having a child, and entering a transitional and potential space (as Winnicottians would say) in order to interpret and create.[16] The "transformative" woman looks to herself and may see a desire to bear a child as "lacking"; the "transitional" woman looks to herself and may see the potential child she desires (however ambivalently) as "missing"; and the "traditional" woman looks to herself and sees both a child and part of her body as lost. All three begin at a slightly different subjective position relative to this "absence" because of their different desires for motherhood. But with the universal social expectation that women should be mothers, regardless of their own personal experience of the "absence," *the idea of absence is always present in their lives as an emptiness, rather than as a generative space.* When there is a shift to childlessness as generative space the childless woman is on the threshold of expanding her experience of female subjectivity.

For the women interviewed, the initiation of a search, or the beginning of a creative labor, was related to what could be called a "structural moment" for their identities. In this moment, a woman's sense of self shifts from a subjective position in which the possibility of motherhood was included in her female identity to an identity configuration in which it was not. Although object-relations and Lacanian theories highlight childhood years in identity development, the adult pathways of childless women reveal the importance of also considering adult developmental issues. Every woman over the course of her reproductive life faces many inquiries regarding her motherhood intentions. Whether she wants them or not these inquiries are discontinuous moments of multiple opportunities to acknowledge to herself and others what it may mean to be a woman who is not a mother. Her answers to these questions often qualitatively change over her lifetime as her sense of self deepens. One 38-year-old woman who had for years responded to these inquiries with, "I just haven't started yet," found herself quite spontaneously at her 20th high school reunion saying for the first time to classmates who asked, "No, I don't have any children," and then going on to share what was significant in her life. She realized from this experience that her delay was a decision and that for her the "twentieth reunion seemed the time to get real."

For many of the traditional women, and for some of the transformative and transitional women, the shift in subjective position regarding her childless state is part of an active mourning process. A 44-year-old woman was reluctantly making her work as a business analyst a larger part of her identity as she moved toward adjusting to her infertility. She realized that she had much more grieving to do and was also aware that only when this mourning was completed would other real "possibilities open up" for her identity.

Without this subjective shift toward another creative labor that can balance the social reflection of woman filled only by the maternal, a childless woman can vaguely feel that something is amiss, or she may actually experience "something missing" from her identity. But with this subjective shift from absence as something missing to absence as creative potential, female identity can feel integrated. The sense that something is amiss (the transformative woman), missing (the transitional woman), or lost (the traditional woman) is redefined.

The 46-year-old transformative woman who was an artist had "wondered if I hadn't had the right hormones." She realized through her emerging art that the feminine takes many forms.

A 43-year-old transitional woman, now a writer, could say she felt at one level that a part of her will always want a child and regret she doesn't have one, and at another level can say that her "stories are kind of like my children."

A 42-year-old traditional woman worked to get over feeling that "something was wrong with me and it wasn't fair." Ultimately she was able to leave her job, which did not carry enough of her sense of identity and values, to devote her time and energy to a nonprofit volunteer organization working toward world peace.

For each of these women reaching their own place meant that the cultural and personal sense of absence they felt about not having a child was not as present in their lives as it was before their psychic process had begun.

Because society has so long associated the feminine with the maternal, it is sometimes difficult to view other developmental paths as anything other than substitutes for that which is "missing." The redefinition of "absence" as "potential space" permits an interpretation of female identity development in which nonmaternal identities are equivalent alternatives to, and not substitutions for, maternal identities.

The childless woman is faced with recurring discontinuous moments of confrontation by others, if not herself, regarding motherhood and her identity. Her own self-confrontation of this issue, if successful, will release whatever fantasies of motherhood she has had, and she will grieve the loss of whatever these fantasies have meant for her identity. This will yield a redistribution of psychic energy within her self, and a reconnecting of her female identity to other linkages of female identification, anchored in her past or present significant relationships with women. Through this process the nascent potential within her own absence will make itself present, and she will be able to approach the "generativity" task of midlife with a creative labor of her own making.[17] Erikson's idea of generativity as a midlife task need not be limited to the raising of one's own children.

Every woman, childless or not, must eventually face the reality that, as Marilyn (Chapter 4) summarized it: "Identity doesn't come from being a mother; it comes from inside. The next half of life is to connect with those aspects in me and [know] there is something inside that will be enough." Women who have been mothers must also face an absence when their children leave home. The woman who is a mother must discover she is more than the presence of her child; the woman who is not a mother must discover she is more than the absence of her child. Female childlessness is not a question of gender identity or concerns regarding a woman's sense of female-ness. The broader question is: how does a woman fulfill her own personal identity (to be a subject with desire) when the prescribed gender role for all women remains tied to their biological capacity for reproduction?

Chapter 5 briefly outlined some of the ways feminists are trying to address the issue of representing specifically female experiences. More linguistic elaboration of the feminine, to which women who are not mothers can make a unique contribution, moves the culture closer to the reality that each gender is complete in its own terms, and permits the realization that both genders are structurally "lacking" identities in the sense that everyone has an unconscious. This makes every identity, male or female, an ongoing dialectical process advocated by such diverse theorists as Lacanian analyst Julia Kristeva and object-relational analyst Tom Ogden.

Gender is certainly a salient category of identity, but it does not have to be exclusive or fixed.[18] Women are not all the same. The developmental pathways of the child-free and child*less* women described here offer evidence that a "normal" female identity can be elaborated beyond the parameters of maternity. Although it seems true that a woman's personal identity develops with less need to separate from her identification with her primary caregiver (mother), there is an important difference between a daughter's identity being in some way similar to her mother's and being exactly the same.

When Luce Irigaray (see Chapter 5) speaks of the lack of a female lineage she is referring to the fact that there has been no social representation of a daughter's female identity as separate from her mother's, because culturally it is assumed that all daughters will take their mother's places. A greater number of childless daughters creates a psychic space in which we can see the meaningful difference between sameness and similarity among women.

A part of this discovery process is the question of female aggression in both its positive and negative aspects.[19] Karen (Chapter 3), who struggled to own her aggression, found that when she could acknowledge it more directly the forward momentum aspect of it increased while the negative aspect of pushing or controlling others decreased. In day-to-day life we see evidence of this in women dealing more directly with anger, competition, envy, and so forth between themselves, rather than denying these aspects of themselves and projecting these traits onto men. Harriet Lerner has noted: "the more we continue to reify and glorify woman's nurturant and caretaking abilities (usually linked to motherhood as a 'separate but equal' line of development), the less likely it is that men will identify and utilize their own competence in this area."[20] This focus also makes it less possible for women to legitimately lay claim to their own needs for autonomy and separate competencies (developments associated with positive uses of aggression) without risking their female identity.

Conclusion

Psychoanalytically oriented feminists are beginning to focus on the capacity for mutuality between mother and infant; thus psychological theory is beginning to take the vicissitudes of each mother's unique personality into account.[21] Mothers have always had, and will always have, maternal ambivalence, and mothers have certainly always had many other desires besides mothering, whether or not familial or societal acceptance or validation of these desires was present. Mother's multifaceted personality, not just her "good" or "bad" mothering, has an impact on her child's evolving female identity. Recognition and acceptance of mother's multifaceted personality, and the realization that all of these aspects of a mother's identity are part of the identification process, indicate how a child's female identity can evolve normally from identifications with mother and yet not include motherhood as the primary determinant of that identification. The lives of the women interviewed show that the mother–daughter relationship has many points of identification that are not exclusively tied to the maternal function. Some changes in social context have resulted in greater expression of these nonmaternal desires in the different lives of their daughters who do not become mothers. Many are, in effect, acting on unconscious identifications with these aspects of their mothers. It is only by elaborating aspects of mother's personality apart from her maternal behavior and acknowledging the normal and diversifying influences of those aspects on the young girl's developing sense of self that our theories will expand beyond the reinforcement of dichotomized gender roles.

The lives of childless women add something to our perspective on the early relationship of mother and daughter. Despite the emphasis on father in Lacanian theory regarding the development of language and its critical role in forming human identity, infant research shows the mother's voice and language to be a formative factor before and after birth and long before the oedipal period. Certainly how mother unconsciously and consciously communicates her attitudes and allegiance to cultural rules regarding selfhood, gender, sexuality, and so forth will facilitate or impede her daughter's acceptance of a female identity that does not include motherhood. But the mother's voice is not the only significant female voice that may influence a girl's development. As previously mentioned a woman "in the flesh" who lives a full life apart from motherhood can have a significant impact on a girl child's capacity to imagine herself having a future that does not include motherhood.

If there were more visible examples of alternative lifestyles, would there be even more child-free women in succeeding generations? Perhaps, perhaps not; but this is not the nodal point. The childless women who successfully transform a culturally prescribed absence in their identities into a creative space are unlinking the necessity of motherhood from a fulfilling female identity. Regardless of the numbers of women who do not become mothers in the future, their continued presence and increased acknowledgment will contribute to a greater comfort with a "real space" between women and the acceptance of women as women—mothers or not.

7

The Gendered
View of Identity:
Limitations and Possibilities

All human individuals, as a result of their bisexual disposition
of cross inheritance, combine in themselves both masculine
and feminine characteristics, so that pure masculinity and
femininity remain theoretical constructions of uncertain content.

—Sigmund Freud

Throughout this book I have used the terms "traditional,"
"transitional," and "transformative" women to suggest that
women who are not mothers are both different from and similar to
one another. Yet virtually all of these women have historically been
viewed by society as in some way empty. In psychological terms,
these women have received projections of absence or deviancy from
others in society. Only recently are they beginning to be viewed in
ways that imply something other than a sense of deficiency. There
are also similarities in the way society views childless women and
society's perceptions of "the other woman" in a domestic triangle.
Both are often devalued, yet at the same time both can be envied
because they are believed to possess qualities that the woman as
mother lacks (freedom, sexuality, power).

In the absence of alternative perspectives from which to view
herself, the childless woman, especially the traditional woman, may

identify with the ideas of emptiness or deviancy and make them her own. A number of these women spoke of feeling somehow damaged and not fully women in their own minds because they had not had a child. However, to the degree that a childless woman has internalized a different and more positive perspective, she will not accept these views or projections, and will be a source of disorientation to others. This is most often true among the transformative women who are more likely to say, as did one 40-year-old woman, "There's nothing in me that has to have a child to feel like a woman."

In addition to these women functioning to disrupt an equation of female identity = motherhood, they also function as a "third" in definitions of gender and gender roles. As discussed in Chapters 5 and 6, a "third term" serves to make a space or break between two—mother–infant, a woman–her childless state, and so forth.[1] To begin deconstructing a hierarchical relationship between any two categories, the first step is to revalue the subordinate category; in the case of gender this would involve positively revaluing women to counteract their negative associations with "lack."[2] (This has been one project of 20th-century feminism.) The second step in this process is to introduce a "third term," called an "undecideable," between the two categories. This term is called an "undecideable" because it cannot be assimilated into either of the original two categories; it makes yet another hierarchical arrangement more difficult to establish. (Of interest here for its gender implications is that deconstruction is a process that is never complete, but one that is continually ongoing or becoming.) As the "undecideable," women who are not mothers are neither traditional females nor traditional males. As a third element they are destabilizing our binary arrangement of gender definition and traditional gender roles. Adrienne Harris has amplified this view:

> Gender may in some contexts be as thick and reified, as plausibly real as anything in our character. At other moments, gender may seem porous and insubstantial. Furthermore, there may be multiple genders or embodied selves. For some individuals these gendered experiences may feel integrated, ego-syntonic. For others, the gender contradictions and alternatives seem dangerous and frightening, and so are maintained as splits in the self, dissociated part–objects.[3]

The childless woman clearly does not fulfill the usual gender role society prescribes for women (that of mother). By having a fulfilling life without motherhood she exposes a mistaken assumption of traditional gender roles—that motherhood is the only proper or natural role for women. In reality there are significant flaws in the traditional gender role arrangement for many women, because it is based on an incomplete view of women's nature and an equation of gender identity with personal identity. As a bearer of Other, nonmaternal female energy—an energy that asserts gender and sexual parity, the woman who is not a mother highlights inequality issues between men and women on many levels.

An expanded view of femaleness that would create a more viable place for women who aren't mothers would necessarily alter concepts of gender identity for maleness. Motherhood has been the standard by which society defines adult women; it is also the yardstick against which early male identity is defined. Because mothers are still the primary caretakers in early childhood, and traditional fathers are generally unavailable as consistent role models during the first years of gender identity development, young boys, in separating from mother, link their identities with trying to be and do the opposite of mother (woman). Masculine qualities are originally defined through the process of negation of feminine qualities. The elaboration of the masculine identity retains this reactive foundation even when positive male attributes are or may be added later. The result of this kind of gender identity development process is that a greater proportion of gender identity disorders occur among boys and men than among girls and women.[4]

Women who are not mothers threaten society with the loss of the presumed adult identity for women. By not ever becoming mothers and invalidating by their very presence the universality of this restricted female identity, they may also seem to undermine the bases of gender identity for men. This subtle, and perhaps deeper threat, helps explain why patriarchal society seems to have a stake in keeping the childless woman as the "invisible woman," particularly when she elects her childless state with scant signs of anguish or deviance. Men who strongly identify with being the opposite of women-mothers will find these new women destabilizing. (Women whose identities are also firmly attached to the woman-mother identity need sameness rather than similarity in their relationship with women and will also have trouble finding a way to connect meaningfully with the childless woman.) Men who unconsciously accept the concept of woman-mother and attempt to project this attitude onto the women who aren't mothers will often find their projections unaccepted, sliding off them as if off teflon. This may result in exaggerated stereotypical male behavior in an attempt to gain solid footing in the encounter. Alternatively, they may avoid or disavow her real existence altogether.

This avoidance or disavowal might be thought of in terms of the fear some children may have when first encountering a snake. Because they have learned that living things that move have legs, the sinuous and legless movement of the snake is initially frightening. After they can accommodate their ideas about "things that move" and the way that things move to include the special movement of the snake, their fear subsides and curiosity and interest can take its place. Perhaps this same kind of accommodation of perception can take place regarding women who are not mothers. When women who are not mothers occupy sufficient space in society to be viewed as other than deviant, the concept of women may shift to accommodate these nonmaternal identities in thought and language.

Childless women embody a different kind of female energy that represents a "bodily" basis for the entrance of female "signifiers" besides maternal ones into the collective language of our culture. They bring with their female experience an alternative reading of Freud's "anatomy is destiny." This is possible because they are indeed doing positive things with their lives outside of motherhood, but also because they are psychically negating the equivalency that daughter = (is the same as) mother, thereby providing alternative metaphors for the feminine.

Psychoanalysis explains that psychic representation only becomes possible when the object (or person) is itself missing or somehow negated. Without absence there is no reason for representation to develop, because the object is always present.[5] (In a story Freud told about his grandson, in mother's absence the boy played a game of throwing a spool of thread out of the crib and then pulling it back, saying "Fort" when throwing and "Da" when pulling it back. Freud explained that in this game his grandson was learning to symbolically represent and deal with his mother's goings [Fort] and comings [Da]. Through the repetitive game, the boy both acknowledged his mother's absence and negated it through substituting the spool, going and coming, using language [Fort, Da] to represent it.) If all daughters are or become mothers how can we imagine them as anything else?

Only recently have there been enough daughters who, by not becoming mothers, are negating the equation of woman = mother; they make it glaringly apparent that something is missing in our definitions of "woman" because there is no valid place for them in existing psychological theory. Only with the awareness of this absence does the possibility emerge for other symbolic representations or signifiers of femaleness to take shape. Women who *choose* not to become mothers are an especially transformative element in society now because they make it necessary for "woman" to be symbolically represented by something "other" than maternity.

Technological advances in the areas of fertility research in the past decade have also introduced an uncertainty with regard to our societal assumptions regarding women and motherhood. The inherent paradox here is that whereas society has devoted a great deal of energy and research time to increase the procreative capacity of women, these new technologies have also had the unforeseen consequences of helping to fragment the very stereotype (woman as mother) that these efforts in part have attempted to reinforce.

Procreative technology has been dismantling, if not redefining, motherhood by splitting maternal functions into such distinctions as birth mother, surrogate mother, ovum mother, womb mother, adoptive mother, even the role of co-mother in lesbian families.[6] Prior to these distinctions paternity could always be doubted and debated, but maternity was obvious and incontrovertible. With procreative technology, the meaning of motherhood is no longer stable and well defined. This uncertainty also functions to introduce a psychic "space" wherein additional signifiers of female identity may emerge into the culture. There is little doubt that procreative research and services will continue to grow as women continue to marry at later ages and expand the boundaries of their genetic fertility by delaying childbearing.[7] This burgeoning research will result in even more shifts in the meaning of female and male gender roles.

Many people in our society view the trends of procreative technology and more child-free women, with their shattering of the unitary definition of woman = mother, as dangerous and threatening. As reproduction becomes further removed from biological function and there are a significant number of women who are not mothers, it becomes increasingly evident that what a woman, a man, or a parent is "supposed to be" is really our own social construction rather than innate biological destiny. Given that gender refers to all the symbolic meanings *we attach* to anatomical sexual difference, the realization that women and men are actually *made and not born* provokes tremendous anxiety. This awareness creates uncertainty about what we as women or men "are supposed" to be and do.[8] It should come as no surprise that some people feel threatened by both procreative technologies and childless women, and will mount concerted efforts to shore up the status quo of traditional sex roles—which essentially means keeping women in their places as mothers.

Feminism itself has diversified in the last decade in part over the issues raised by procreative technology and its meaning for motherhood. At times there seems to be a tendency to decry the differences among women implicit in issues such as surrogate motherhood. It may be more useful to welcome these differences as a needed change, a greater differentiation of the female voice, because the feminist movement struggles to overcome stereotypical definitions. Perhaps these different female voices can be imagined as a woman's chorus trying to join an ongoing concert hitherto composed solely of male voices.

A hopeful way of conceiving of 20th-century feminism, along with cycling through the kind of "backlash" Susan Faludi[9] writes about, is that collectively, we as a society are engaged in what Donald Winnicott described as the infant's necessary developmental process of destroying the omnipotent mother inside her or his mind to discover the real mother outside.[10] According to Winnicott, only by discovering the mother as a real subject can the infant relate to her, develop an authentic individual identity, and have the capacity for mutuality in relationship. Perhaps 20th-century American society is, at one level, attempting to "destroy" the omnipotent *unconscious* representation of woman (woman as all-giving or all-denying mother) so that real external women in their diverse subjective experiences, unique gifts, and fallibilities, may be *consciously* discovered, as Winnicott suggested, and related to mutually.

Childless women as "Other women" may be thought of as figures bridging the gap between the pragmatic–political perspective of the majority of American feminists and the more philosophical perspective of many European feminists. Childless women expose as illusion the idea that "woman" has existed historically as an authentic Other for men, when in reality she has been portrayed as his lesser opposite. In terms of the complementary psychoanalytic theories discussed in earlier chapters, the Europeans, influenced by Lacan, emphasize the illusion of the self as one, or whole, and also the relative dearth of female experience in patriarchal language. The Americans, influenced by the British school of object-relations theory, emphasize the significance and necessity of illusion in the mother–infant dyad for the grounding of an authentic, coherent self, whether female or male, as well as the need for practical social changes for women.

Childless women, by their increased presence, help establish female identity in both pragmatic–political and intellectual terms. The meaning of "woman" is no longer collapsed into or limited by motherhood; all daughters do not take their mothers' places. Because these women give form and substance to a vertical relationship between women (the daughter no longer has a continuous identity with mother achieved by taking her place, i.e., herself becoming a mother), they make possible a more horizontal relationship between women, where differences can be more fully acknowledged in negative as well as positive ways.[11]

The common field of play for both American and European feminism is the role of language in human identity and subjectivity. The common task then becomes to determine how language, in all its inherent ambiguity, can be used to create alternative identities outside the traditional and expected identity configurations for women.[12]

Thus the project of modern feminism, despite the differing views of how to approach it, is to bring more female experience into the net of language, which though always falling short of reflecting full human experience, remains central in constructing psychological theory, social policy, and laws regulating the human (and more

often the female) "body." It is all we have. This is essential if
"Woman" is to truly exist as a real Other (and not just remain a male
negation or fantasy), as a female subject with her own desires.
Increasingly, women who are not mothers are making a marked
contribution to this arena. Women who are able to utilize their
childlessness, a socially prescribed absence, as a third term to
facilitate personal adult development are simultaneously expanding the meaning of female subjectivity itself and are disrupting fixed
and traditional gender roles.

These women, either willingly or reluctantly, are at the
forefront of the shifting perceptions to which our advances in
reproductive freedom, feminism, and procreative research have
brought us. They stand at the threshold of exploring new ways of
understanding women and men. Their increasing numbers and
their development of adult identities without motherhood prompt
us to focus on and reevaluate our perceptions regarding the
relationship of woman to her womb, relationships between sexes,
and the inner space of the unconscious self. Each of these could be
seen as representing a liminal space—a space at the threshold of
greater understanding and appreciation of women, men, and the
human condition.

Metaphorizing the Body

The child-free or childless woman provides a reinterpretation of the
feminine that is less tied than in the past to the female's physical
capacity of reproduction. Society has generally preferred to ignore
or minimize this metaphorical meaning.

Freud said "anatomy is destiny." It is not necessary to restrict
our interpretation of these words to their literal meaning. Women
need not necessarily concretize the metaphorical possibilities of
their womb space to the biological meaning of childbearing, nor
need the words representing "woman" be restricted to reproduction per se. The varied lives of women who aren't mothers support
the idea that motherhood is more of a culturally embedded
mandate than a biological or psychological mandate. The female
body, the womb space (specifically, woman space) can be viewed as
a generalized creative metaphor of holding and bringing forth.
Rather then limiting women to their reproductive function, the
womb could be seen as a metaphor for the holding of all our creative

seeds and the birthing of generative possibilities, as a way of being that could be termed a "feminine creative posture."

To describe this more fully, the womb is a liminal space existing at the threshold between real and symbolic offspring. Many of the women interviewed perceived that creative work had an important role in developing and sustaining their adult identity. These women are creating additional metaphors (symbolic offspring, if you will) that reflect female themes of interconnection and embedded identity rather than metaphors of solitude and conquest, which are typically masculine. A feminine creative posture might be such as Marilyn, the transformative woman of Chapter 4, described it:

> *I think of the feminine as something which is coming from the unconscious, or coming from inside. There is the element of having to open yourself up to what is given rather than deciding want you want. You take what comes. I think that is a very feminine capacity for experience. The masculine is more of "I'm going to decide what I want and go after it." The feminine is, "I'm going to open myself up to what might or might not be there and discover what it is."*

This interpretive act or position holds the Other as always implicitly present, as the "child" that could be possible. This interpretive position need not be tied exclusively to women, it is only that the female body seems to carry the metaphor of self *and* other more readily.

Opening the female womb to its metaphoric potential enables a woman to be seen as complete unto herself in the same way as a man is. This shift also opens another symbolic view of the male's erect penis—different from its usual symbolism of difference, separateness, and oneness. In extending for the other, the erect penis also carries the metaphor of self and other in a different emotional way than the womb. The womb may hold or "take in" the other, while the penis reaches to engage the other or penetrate the other's subjective space. Rather than viewing the penis as penetrating the other's subjective space, and viewing the womb as a passive container, an alternate metaphor may view the womb as a active embracer of the other, and the erect penis as a means of reaching toward and fully accepting the embrace.

Women's lives that lie beyond the parameters of motherhood,

but are woven within the context of relationships, challenge the unfortunate overemphasis on maternity in psychological theories of the relationship model of female development. Focus on the gender-based capacity (reproduction) obstructs the possible reinterpretation of the metaphors of human individuation from ones of complete separateness and autonomy (commonly represented by men) to metaphors of interconnection and mutuality, which more often represent women's experience, mothers or not. With regard to human evolution, exploration needs to be expanded to include the question of whether, in addition to reproduction, our common survival requires more of what has traditionally been labeled feminine relatedness, but is in fact an essential need of both genders.

The absence attributed to women who are not mothers, because they do not bear children from their wombs, may be reframed as a lack of cultural emphasis on the feminine and the use of feminine metaphors per se, as well as a missing interpretation of the male body as a source for metaphors of connection. What has actually been culturally absent has been the naming and representation of nonmaternal female experience.

Ecological and other threatening conditions are increasingly requiring nations to remain connected beyond political boundaries to maintain their welfare. As separateness and autonomy give way to the need for connectedness in individual as well as global contexts, the cultural recognition of female experiences and female ways of shaping these experiences (within and beyond maternity) becomes more and more relevant for human survival and less the idiosyncratic project of feminists. A feminine interpretive position of psychically holding the Other as always implicitly present in one's judgments, contrasted with making judgments based on what is perceived as abstractly right, is becoming imperative at a global level.

Western society has traditionally devalued the meaning of relationships in developing and sustaining identity after childhood, focusing instead on individual development of the autonomous self. When there is more societal recognition that a coherent self can only be discovered, developed, and sustained by relationships with others throughout life, the possibility is opened for developing a day-to-day ethic rooted in the context of meaningful relatedness to others.[13]

The Space Between the Sexes

Does the space between the sexes need always to be conceived of as a battle zone because of inherent power issues? Power struggles have historically been linked to sexual differences between men and women; with men taking their own biology as the standard from which women are then judged to be incomplete. This has meant that the concept of difference has become unnecessarily wedded to a chronic condition of inequality for women. The woman who has chosen the developmental path of motherhood has, by her need to devote time and energy to childraising (a reality despite the protestations of equality in childrearing) placed herself in the position of needing support, but this does not have to mean whole-scale inequality. Is the woman denied the ability to bear a child relegated to a substitute feminine identity? What of the woman who chooses not to have a child? Is she denying the reality of her biologically destined, inherently less-powerful self or is rather choosing an equally valid, equally feminine course.

Many women, mothers or not, say they want from a man a *different but equal* partner to journey with.[14] This kind of relationship seems at least partially linked at this historical time to the separation of female identity from motherhood. Having a child always increases the undertow of socialized sex roles. When a woman is capable of financial independence and is not in the role of mother, it is easier for her to develop an equal relationship with a man. When neither member in a relationship is a parent, both women and man are a little freer to wonder why each should be expected to do and be certain ways just because of their sexual difference.

The road map of traditional gender roles seems to make the process of relationship easier to navigate. The absence of the dimension of parenting in a relationship opens another door on femininity and masculinity—one that beckons both woman and man toward exploration of the meaning of gender and of each other's personal identity with fewer constraints—but with more uncertainty. This uncharted journey is a bittersweet process; it is an effort of both partners reaching for moments of mutual understanding amidst the shifting sands of gender role ambiguity. When mutuality is reached, even if fleetingly, conditions are created that enhance a kind of dialogue between them that differs considerably from the usual conversation between the sexes where the man is seen as having greater power in the relationship and in the world simply because he has a penis.

This journeying relationship between a woman and man is a step away from the personal identity rigidly encased in the gender stereotypes. It is a step toward appreciating and learning about the fluidity and uniqueness of individual differences without the distortion of gender-specific lenses. This kind of relating make the space between the sexes less a gender-related and defined battle zone and more of a liminal space. In this space, the threshold is the meaning of sexual difference that can be explored and questioned within the framework of each person's needs and desires, rather than being dictated by social rules for female and male behavior. A similar kind of liminal space can also exist in lesbian, gay, and coparenting couples who develop primary relationships outside the usual script of traditional gender roles. In each of these nontraditional relationships the partners must create their own rules for living because, by definition, they cannot fit into stereotypical gender roles. Coparenting couples are stepping outside the usual gender roles of woman as primary parent and man as primary provider. In all these nontraditional relationships the distinction between personal–individual differences and gender differences are apparent.

"Childless" Women, Absence, and the Illusion of Wholeness

In their lack of identification with what has historically been the central feature of female identity (motherhood), childless women are an apt metaphor of our postmodern times, a period in which philosophy and psychoanalytic theory have brought to our attention the de-centered or divided nature of the self.[15]

The postmodernist perspective has focused on the inherent discontinuities and gaps in our life experience and identities. These "gaps" are related to the presence of the unconscious and the limited capacity of language to fully express our personal experiences. In less technical terms, the postmodern chapter of history opened at the place of "absent or missing places" in human identity; childless women mark this place. What does this really mean?

We have yet to appreciate the meaning of the unconscious, which is integral to each individual. For the most part we attempt to deny either its existence or its importance. Even among those whose theories presuppose its existence, there is often little real recognition of its profound implications. This individual denial cannot help but have an impact on our social structures; many believe that continuing in a state of psychic denial carries global risk. Knowledge has increased exponentially, yet the problems of human relationship, on a family or a nationwide scale, have not diminished. More knowledge does not seem to be the answer; more wisdom, and a further understanding and acceptance of the self, may be what we need.

In the manner that childless women do not only portray emptiness related to absence, but an alternative form of female or human fullness, the absent part of the self, the unconscious, can also be a source of information for the conscious part of the individual or group identity. This absent part of our selves (absent only from awareness) speaks, dreams, and acts through us in moments that can be illuminating, delightful, disturbing, and unsettling. It is the place within us that is also a well from which both our desires and creativity spring. The liminal quality of this absent space is that threshold between meaning and nonmeaning. By accepting its reality, it is possible to take something seemingly disconnected and meaningless that appears from the absent unconscious and forge something meaningful and useful from it in the present.[16]

The psychic encounter of a woman and the absence of a child often occurs in midlife, but the midlife crossing accentuates a woman's own particular identity evolution, *apart from* as well as including the issues of childlessness. For both men and women, the midlife crossing is a ripe opportunity (though not necessarily the only one) for reframing what is missing or absent in one's identity as "potential space" to be explored. Relatedness to one's absence is an identity model that is relevant here, and available for all.

Midlife is a time of inner confrontation with those childhood identifications and illusions that have somehow carried us halfway through our lives. It is a time of facing one's own misrecognitions (as Lacan would put it) based on our identifications with others, and facing our fantasies of who we thought we might be at midlife.[17] An essential task of this midlife period, a task in which all the women interviewed were either involved or at the brink of entering, is to find, via inner psychic confrontation (sometimes through psychotherapy), something authentic among the debris and the trophies garnered from earlier identifications—identifications always assumed to be ourselves. This holds true for females and males, whether childless or not.

In the individuation process, as Carl Jung called the process of moving toward, yet never reaching, psychic wholeness, each person must encounter what is or has been essentially absent in her or his own life and how this absence is related to what has been present in life.[18] At the threshold of midlife a dialogue between the conscious (present) part of one's self and the unconscious (absent) part often begins in earnest; we sort through those of our dreams that have been fulfilled, those that have not, and why (for ourselves or for someone else). Through actively engaging in this dialogue women and men, childless or not, will become more able to face the developmental tasks of the second half of life, and come to terms with the inevitability of the final absence—death itself.

The adult pathway of the woman who does not have a child merely makes more visible this particularly human challenge—that of developing a more conscious adult identity by accepting, indeed, actively engaging with the absent (unconscious) parts of the self. Absence, then, is "potential space"; its engagement is a creative possibility that all individuals are challenged to accept.

One interpretation of the value of dichotomized gender roles is that the strict definition of what it means to be male and female permits the separation of sexually ascribed attributes to maintain a separation of conscious and unconscious processes, and thereby maintain a denial of the existence and meaning of the unconscious to each individual human being. Those processes generally thought of as unconscious are more closely allied with attributes generally described as feminine (consider, for example, women's intuition); the more conscious, reality-based, activity-oriented processes are more closely allied with attributes generally described as masculine (for example, the logical, clear-speaking woman who is said to "think like a man").

Society has used complementary traditional gender roles in part to deny the profound implications of the discontinuity of human experience. By ascribing all aspects of identity either to men or women, based on gender differences, we deny the conflictual reality that all men and women are divided human beings living with the unpredictable effects of unconscious processes, attempting to sustain the illusion of the completely known self. The placing of "the unconscious" in the female stereotype and making it conscious but separate and devalued, avoids the need to deal with the reality that both men and women are subject to the unpredictable (and at times undesireable) effects of unconscious processes and the inevitable conclusion that human identity (male or female) and relationships are always somewhat precarious and discontinuous. Maintaining this illusion requires the collusion of both women and men; but the illusion is maintained at greater expense to women.

A model of identity that perceives gender and gender roles as fluid, discontinuous, and as a dialectic between conscious and unconscious, rather than as singular and fixed concepts, would provide the opportunity for a greater variety of personal and social roles to be held by both women and men. Because this model would not serve the purpose of maintaining a false sense of cohesive individual identity, it lends itself to the possibility that human beings will be able to embrace the inherent discontinuity of human identity, and holds the promise of a more *real* encounter with both self and the other on an individual and group level. As each person begins to more fully accept and relate to her or his own inner unconscious and the partiality of identity that this implies, a mutual dialogue between two authentic human beings becomes possible.[19]

The idea of an authentic self does not necessarily imply wholeness or continuity, but does imply some coherence. Accepting the partiality of human experience at every level of personal identity (including gender and sexuality) frees us from the need to establish gender-based roles that maintain a fixed illusion of wholeness. We provide a space in which both women and men can explore the meaning of the coherence of an identity freer from arbitrary gender-role constraints.

Childless women, as women, but certainly as "other women," call attention to the undervalued presence of the unconscious, that something absent from our everyday awareness, the Other to our waking conscious self. If they are to establish a positive atypical female identity, these women must address the paradox that in the idea of absence (having no children) there is also presence and fullness. In the process of dealing with the paradox of absence these women offer an alternative model of identity, one that rejects the view of "absence" by transforming it through relatedness; a relatedness to their own Other. Childless women as a metaphor for the dialectic of absence and presence in human identity are indeed holding a third position in our gender role schema; they are not being the lack, the position women have traditionally held, nor are they denying the lack and claiming wholeness, the traditional position held by men in patriarchal societies. As the different identities of childless women receive more social recognition and acceptance, their process will aid in legitimizing a model of identity embracing the discontinuity of the self; a model of identity that acknowledges that unconscious processes are part of an individual's or country's life and relationships. Utilizing this "absent space" within us can lead to living life as an ongoing creative project, in which the existence and contributions of both conscious and unconscious processes are more fully acknowledged.[20]

How might we visualize a model of the discontinuous self—this dialectic between absence and presence? In schematic diagrams of self and others used by psychology and psychoanalysis, the image of the circle is commonly employed to represent both self and other. The continuity of the circle's perimeter represents the basic sense of coherence of identity. When the ends of a long, thin strip of paper are connected to make a circle, it is impossible to trace both sides of the circle with a single, uninterrupted line. One side of the circle may be said to represent the conscious, and the other side the unconscious parts of the individual. The circle accurately represents notions of identity that leave unconscious processes outside the picture.

However, German mathematician August Möbius noted that if a thin strip of paper is twisted in the center before its ends connect, what results is a shape that is like a circle, but it is a figure surface on which a single line can be traced to cover both sides of the strip. This describes a dynamic relationship between the inside and the outside of the figure. In tracing the edge of the strip around the circle, at some point the tracing of the *outside* of the circle will become *inside*. The shifting back and forth and the ambiguity between outside and inside provided by the Möbius strip offers a more apt metaphor for individual identity and the dynamic relationship between the conscious and unconscious. There is coherence to this figure, yes, but also a fluidity and discontinuity as well.[21]

A circle can also be the image representing traditional gender roles. The perimeter defining the circle is maleness and all that is within is his creation. Femaleness, all that is outside the perimeter, is left undefinable and unspeakable, except in relation to the circle itself. The Möbius strip in this instance also provides an alternative model of relationship between the sexes. What is inside or outside gender role definitions for each sex shifts dramatically by substituting the metaphor of the Möbius strip, which offers a fluid dialectic between women and men, whereas the circle, in its fixedness, does not.

In psychodynamic terms we could say that the larger group of women who are not mothers applies social and psychic pressure on the Möbius strip to move what has been outside the perimeter of the circle (femaleness in all its multiplicity) to inside, seeking further symbolic and linguistic representation. The Möbius strip is an image better reflecting the fluidity of individual identity and the "uncertain contents" of masculinity and femininity of which Freud spoke.

Inconclusion

A significant challenge in the 21st century will be to legitimize a model of individual and collective identity that is not based on an illusion of wholeness or rightness. Cultural resistance to recognizing the different lives of childless women seems related to the fact that these women lives illuminate the complexity and diversity of human identity.

Women who are not mothers may have been ghettoized in psychological theory because their lives, in so many ways, point out the essential and never-ending dynamic tension underlying the development of a stable identity, particularly the tension of gender and sexuality.[22] Freud himself acknowledged that in any sexual act there are four people participating; both genders are represented psychically (the unconscious identification with both parents) and carried by each individual, regardless of her or his biological gender, into this intimate exchange.[23] (Likewise, the unconscious complement to the individual's expressed sexual orientation is also present in this exchange.) The concrete quality of Freud's comment that "anatomy is destiny," made in later years, belies this earlier understanding, which expressed his intuitive realization that gender and sexual identity are problematic concepts at best. These are difficult areas currently being explored by psychoanalytically oriented feminists.

By living meaningful lives, childless women challenge many of the popular, socially accrued meanings attributed to sexual differences; this makes us uncomfortable. For example the primary relationships of childless women force us to rethink basic ideas about the meaning and interplay of gender and sexuality. We can no longer ignore the fact that female sexuality exists and expresses itself separately from its reproductive function.

The diverse views of gender and sexuality made possible by acknowledging the dialectic between the conscious and the unconscious reveal the multidimensional nature of and possibilities present in human life. But this concept also illuminates the ambiguity, ambivalence, and anxiety of confronting the partiality of human experience—exacted by the existence of the unconscious. As noted previously, dichotomized sex roles help maintain the illusion of the wholeness of human experience, an illusion that is needed for social functioning but not to the extent or degree of rigidity currently existing. The most useful illusion is one that one is aware of maintaining; but those illusions that are maintained without realizing that they are illusions tend to become limiting. The risk of, and resistance to, social recognition of "woman but not mother" derives from the loss of the presumed psychic security that this illusion (unacknowledged as such) perpetuates.

Women who are not mothers indeed reside in a paradoxical realm. They seem to disrupt the boundaries between the sexes, but they also expand the definition and subjectivity of what it means to be a woman. They make us aware that society's rules for gender, sexuality, and other social roles, are in part an attempt to minimize the disruptive effects of the unconscious on our identities. In attempting to screen out the awareness of those unconscious elements of our identities, we constrict the very source of personal creativity. In attempting to screen out of awareness the female identities which do not include motherhood, society constricts the identity development of both women and men. The dichotomous gender roles adopted to sustain an illusion of wholeness have defined the absent (unconscious) aspects of self as female. The childless women of the coming century, in their role as a third term, present the opportunity to reframe absence in such a way that it may be reintegrated less threateningly into, not merely a feminine identity, but a more complete human identity.

The heterogeneous lives and roles of child*less* and child-free women are part of feminism's hope that the 21st century promises something other than fixed gender-roles in futuristic clothing. By receiving the projections of absence and emptiness from others, and returning them altered through their own full lives, these women can underscore the importance for all of being meaningfully related to the "absent" reservoir of the unconscious. These women, defined by society in terms of "something missing," can offer something more. As they take a more prominent place in discussions about gender, they will reveal the nature of woman beyond the maternal function. They offer no answers regarding women or gender, but as women of a transitional time, they issue an invitation to both men and women to enter and explore the absent space within and between themselves—viewing this space not as empty or barren, but as an ambiguous, liminal space, waiting to be creatively filled . . . emptied . . . filled . . . and emptied again.

8

Women But Not Mothers

Much of the feminine is aptly described by an analytic term coined by Christopher Bollas, the "unthought known." Female experience is better known as a palpable presence in our society rather than by being verbally articulated and differentiated.[1] As I noted in previous chapters it is the continuing project of many women today to bring more of the female experience into language in terms other than those that define women in opposition to men. With this in mind, at the conclusion of all the interviews I began to wonder how it might be possible to speak of the experience of women who aren't mothers in other than theoretical terms. This led me to begin to search for a known story or metaphor that could at least partially frame the experience of these women.

My search took me to the library of the C. G. Jung Institute of San Francisco. A friend and I spent hours among the shelves of books, seeking a myth or legend of a woman who had not been a mother. I was looking for representation of female diversity that might have existed prior to the patriarchal times of the familiar Greek goddesses. The search ended when I found the legend of Lilith—a creation story of the first woman and man. Other stories or myths doubtless also offer a framework, but here was a place to begin to think and speak about female experience from a different perspective.

The creation myth of Lilith can be used as a metaphorical frame for aspects of female identity and subjectivity that have long been present in the unconscious of every woman, and that women have historically struggled to voice and claim as their own. This legend reveals some of the roots of the negative portrayals of women who aren't mothers and provides understanding of the incipient social threat these women pose as the "other woman." It also points us toward a direction for integrating this "other" kind of female energy. Here is the story of Lilith.

According to legend, Lilith was the first woman, created by God from the matter of earth, like Adam, the first man.[2] Lilith and Adam began to argue over who would "lie beneath" the other during sex. Lilith soon became aware that neither was listening to the other, so she uttered the name of God and "flew into the air of the word," running away to reside by the sea.

Adam complained to God that Lilith had run away. God then sent three angels to bring her back, saying that if she refused, she must be prepared to sacrifice 100 of her sons each day. Lilith refused. She said that she was destined to weaken infants (boys for 8 days and girls for 20 days) unless they were protected by the names of the three angels who had come for her or by the image of God. In later elaborations of the legend, Lilith, on some of her return visits from the Red Sea, would visit men in their sleep, bringing them wet dreams.

This creation story of woman and man was later amended to name Eve as the first woman; it is this amended version that appears in the book of Genesis. Eve, being made from the rib of Adam, begins on less than equal footing. Eve's single expression of Lilith's independent, equal nature has catastrophic consequences. It is Eve who first bites the forbidden apple of knowledge, resulting in the couple's expulsion from Eden and a lifetime of painful childbirth. Lilith embodies female characteristics that were essentially deleted from the mythic roots of the womanhood portrayed by Eve. Lilith, who is made of earth like Adam, manifests woman's difference in equal terms instead of woman's difference being defined in opposite and lesser terms than man.

This legend also reveals what the less-than-desirable consequences are when woman is cut off from a mutual relationship and must live in a patriarchal society that denies her equality. When there is lack of acceptance and support for a woman's independent impulses the effects upon herself and others are likely to be distorted. Lilith births her own kind of children (not born of man) but is forced to sacrifice 100 of them each day—her own creative contributions are constantly diminished, as it were. In these circumstances she also carries a destructive potential, perhaps associated with a malignant envy, toward other women's children. Because her sexuality is denied she must cloak her natural desire in the folds of night, to seek satisfaction from unavailable partners.

On the other side of the coin, Lilith suggests a direction to pursue regarding the expansion of female identity. Her legend illustrates both repression and the importance of language in constructing human subjectivity. Lilith spoke the name of God in the moment before she left Adam. Considering the role of language in human subjectivity (see Chapter 5) one could interpret Lilith's speaking of God's name as empowering her own destiny. Did not God recognize the validity of her claim to her own subjectivity by not forcing her to return to Adam?

In old testament stories related to Lilith, it was said that, in her surreptitious returns from the Red Sea, she promised to forsake her evil ways toward whomever they were directed if that person would call her by one or all of her fourteen names. This seems to be an attempt, through the use of language, to legitimate female subjectivity. I would like to suggest that when the feminine has more access to conscious "names" (words/identities) other than motherhood, the apparently threatening aspects of the childless women, who, in part, bear the repressed and disavowed aspects of Lilith, will be experienced as less threatening and destructive to others (and at times themselves).

A conscious remembrance and removal of the repression of female empowerment and female desire, as metaphorized in the story of Lilith, is needed. Many women of the twentieth century have been and are engaged in this effort. Yet women who are mothers are not really required to integrate the energy that Lilith symbolizes into their female identities. They can remain identified with the female energy of Eve, although their lives will be less vital without this integration. However, women who are not mothers must reintegrate the nonmaternal female energy symbolized by Lilith into their female identities if they are to forge a positive adult identity; they cannot include within their self-definitions the identity of woman as mother, together with the socially assumed meanings that this role implies. If they do not integrate this independent and creative energy, they are left with a damaged or deviant sense of self.

The "traditional" woman, involuntarily a nonmother, confronts the task of letting in the Lilith part of herself, so to speak, in order to transform her female identity. The woman who discovers she is infertile does not become childless overnight. The traditional woman illustrates most clearly the primary dynamic of mourning— of a lost opportunity to develop an adult self in which mother is very primary to her identity. She must undergo a process of becoming, however reluctantly, a different woman. This is a process she experiences gradually over time in discontinuous moments of psychic change. In certain catalyzing moments (sometimes prompted by a casual stranger's question about children) something inside of her shifts to re-form her adult female identity. The traditional woman must open herself to the Lilith side of her nature, so that her life unfolds not as a substitute for motherhood but on another equally meaningful pathway. She must broaden her identification with the feminine beyond Eve to include aspects not attached to maternity. As she does this, her life will take on a different character as seen in the lives in Martina and Diane of Chapter 2. Although each found other places for their maternal energies, they also reached for and developed aspects of themselves that were not identified with maternity. Had they been unable to accept the unrealizability of motherhood and to relinquish or reorient that self-definition, their lives would most likely be pervaded with bitterness, disappointment, and/or a sense of failure.[3]

"The finality of my childlessness came gradually," one 43-year-old woman said. By this she meant there were multiple points at which she absorbed the meaning and implications of this knowledge for her life, while shifting her energy and attention to other relationships and activities. Another 38-year-old woman said she had to overcome the sense of being a "defective woman," and moved toward a career in homeopathic medicine, which included caring for others, an element important to her. Another 47-year-old woman who had tried many infertility treatments spoke of a very real and prevalent problem. She said her own process of shifting her female identity would have been easier and less prolonged if "society didn't make women feel so abnormal if they don't have children." For these women, more than for the "transitional" or "transformative" women, the melding of their own maternal wishes with the social expectation that all women should be or would want to be mothers can be difficult to differentiate, and this can serve to prolong their grieving.

The situation for the transitional woman is bit different. The transitional woman, childless by delay, is actively struggling to integrate two aspects of her female identity, woman as mother and woman as something else. (If this struggle were thought of in terms of Eve and Lilith energies rather than female or male sex roles, the struggle would probably be experienced differently and look different to others viewing her conflict.) The transitional woman, as seen in the lives of Karen and Jane in Chapter 3, experiences the tension and conflict of multiple desires. Her pathway in life offers a look into the ubiquitous human dilemma of moving between different subjective positions in regard to one's own unfolding life. This dialectic concerns the shift back and forth between just being immersed in one's life of the moment versus making the attempt to give meaning to these life experiences by interpretation, as amplified in Chapter 6. It is through this process that one's identity evolves. The mourning prominent for the traditional woman may be more variable for the transitional woman, depending on the extent to which the potential identity of mother was a part of her unique, unconscious, personal identity. A 43-year-old woman commented that she saw herself as having ridden the waves of the social movements of the 1960s and 1970s into the 1980s without much self-reflection. She then began to step back from her immersion in the external events of her life to begin to wonder about how her wish for a child actually fit into her pursuit of becoming a freelance photographer, and how both of these desires fit with her current status as a woman alone.

In part, transitional women show the struggle and sacrifice inherent to every life, although, of course, the content of the struggle and sacrifice is always individual. Struggling to reconcile and fulfill both maternal and nonmaternal desires, and faced with the reality that childbearing is very unlikely or impossible, she must strive to consciously accept and understand her particular circumstances, letting go of her identification with her womb as the place to nourish a child so that another kind of creative child may be born. If this nonmaternal creative labor is already present (as with the photographer just mentioned) its true significance to her identity must be validated. In this act, the female energy of Lilith is activated, so to speak, and her different pathway becomes clearer. Both Karen and June had to become more conscious of their creative and career striving in order to release and make use of their assertive energy. One 44-year-old woman expressed something essential about the transitional woman's dilemma when she said, "I always thought of myself as having a child, but someday was always a long time away. . . . There's a part of me that could have had a child and been happy with that, but I guess it isn't as big as the part of me that felt not having a child was the right for me. There's been a lot of tension between these two parts of myself."

In contrast to the traditional or transitional woman, the transformative woman, by choice not a mother, is aligned earlier in life with Lilith's, rather than Eve's, female energy. She is drawn to a quest outside of the territory of motherhood. Identifying, following, and engaging herself in the realization of her nontraditional interests may make her feel very much like Lilith—a woman alone, if not in exile. As such, she realizes the importance of connecting with others who value her difference. She also knows that she bears a certain burden of others' misunderstanding or nonacceptance of a woman choosing a life of her own. One 50-year-old woman discovered this truth early in adulthood when she told her office mates of her plan for a "child-free" life and subsequently became the recipient of anonymous hate mail. Prior to the women's movement it was very difficult to find other women of like mind with whom she could relate and identify. It is easier now for transformative women to find a peer group.[4]

The 42-year-old woman who said her creative self was like "a little ember that somebody blew on and I just had to go with it" is expressing the experience of many transformative women who are simply following the inner call toward an individual life. This life needn't be exceptional, in fact it may be very ordinary, but it is a female life apart from the experience of mothering, which, to some people, still is an extraordinary choice. Today there are "healthy women making healthy choices not to have children but to do something else with their lives," is how one 46-year-old would like others to see it. Perhaps the words that best summarize the transformative women's feelings about their lives are those of a 43-year-old woman who, toward the end of the interview, said: "If I made jigsaw puzzle pieces out of every aspect of my life and I then put them all together, there would not be a big gap in the middle that was somehow the 'unborn child' in my life."

Though all these women who aren't mothers are different in some respects from women who are, they are also similar. When I asked each woman at the end of the interview to imagine herself as an old woman looking back over her life and how she would like to see it, the answers were very revealing. All three groups of women mentioned these themes: the importance of their significant relationships for their happiness and well-being; their wish to enrich the lives of others around them; and a desire to have learned how to enjoy life fully. In addition to these themes, the transitional women said they would want to have the feeling that they had lived a life that was true to becoming themselves. This is not surprising given the dialectic of consciousness demonstrated by this group of women. To the common themes mentioned by all three groups, the transformative women added the hope that a contribution of theirs would somehow be recognized. This wish for recognition poignantly speaks to their wish to be seen as living a valuable life, not just personally, but also socially. It would seem that all these thoughts express the desires of many women today (mothers or not) regarding how they would like to view their lives from the vantage point of old age: to have loved and been loved, to have been a contributing member of their community and been socially acknowledged for it, to have learned how to be playful and enjoy, and last but not least, to have lived an authentic life.

Women who are integrating a version of Lilith's energy into their adult identities and who are also not mothers need not continue to be absent in our society; they need only be named. The legend of Lilith is only one point of departure for thinking and speaking of female experience outside stereotypic notions: It offers a name and range of meaning for womanhood not contained in the Eve legend of Western Judeo-Christian tradition. Other names and words are needed and they will come.

Using "child-free" or "childless by choice" as words to categorize women is inadequate. "Child*less*" or "child-free" still focuses our attention on the identity of woman in terms of attachment to a child; they still define her in relation to mothering rather than as an individual and separate person making choices. Judith from Chapter 4, who had chosen a life of her own, reflected changing reactions to inquiries about whether she had children. Judith used to avoid situations in which the question of children would arise because of her own discomfort with her childless status. Now she notices that some parents who long for a freedom that parenthood does not allow envy her not having any children. Also, her working-through process has enabled her to *shift her experience of what is not in her life to what is in her life* leaving a deficiency model of her womanhood behind.

Whatever future words are used to describe woman and women's experiences need to come from the place of *what is* rather than *what is not*.

During one interview, a 40-year-old woman was reflecting on how much the culture had changed in her lifetime, especially as it related to expanding women's choices in life. She put into words something crucial regarding conceptions of female identity and women's own experience of themselves: "When was the last time you heard a forty-year-old woman described as an old maid? I mean, no one talks that way anymore. And no one thinks of themselves that way anymore."

Language contributes to shaping who we are—women and men. There will come a time in the future when a woman who may or may not be a mother will find herself in a conversation about women's lives and choices and someone, perhaps even she herself, will say: "Well, when was the last time you heard a forty-year-old woman described as childless? I mean, no one talks that way anymore."

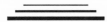

Appendix: Research Data

Summary of Previous Research on Childless Women

Research on women without children has been marred by inconsistency regarding the definition of childlessness. Childless by choice, delay, or infertility, or some combination of these, occurs in the literature, with the assumption that women in each of these categories are similar to women in other categories. In this study the groups are considered separately. Women childless by choice have been identified as "transformative" women; those childless by chance or delay have been called "transitional" women; and the group childless by infertility have been designated "traditional" women.

Many previous studies are also characterized by a limited sampling selection. Most studies have used married, highly educated, Caucasian-American women as subjects. Utilizing only married Caucasian-American women as subjects of study leaves out many other women who are childless and deal with the task of developing a satisfying adult female identity apart from motherhood.

These methodological inadequacies have no doubt contributed to conflicting conclusions about women and childlessness.[1] Mixed definitions of childlessness have also made comparisons among studies difficult. But with these limitations in mind, let us consider some of the findings.

Initial research on almost any minority group (race, class, sexual preference, etc.) often begins by determining if members of that minority are in any way different or more pathological from members of the dominant majority group, generally defining pathology with reference to the majority norm. Psychological research examining childless women has found that women without children have no more psychological disturbance than do women with children.[2] The women who *choose* to remain child-free have been found, however, to value their personal freedom more, to be more autonomous and achievement oriented, and to have a less traditional sex-role orientation than women who are mothers.[3] Women who choose to remain child-free have also been found to be more educated and employed at higher status jobs than are women who are mothers; this corresponds to a common stereotype of childless women as career women.[4]

Although there are many reasons why a woman may choose not to become a mother, the three most frequent reasons women give for choosing a child-free life are: (1) more mobility and greater freedom to pursue other interests because of freedom from childcare responsibilities; (2) a more satisfactory marital relationship; and (3) career considerations.[5] Also the quality of primary relationships among voluntarily childless women appears different from those of married women with children. In comparative studies, childless couples have been found to report more couple interaction, higher marital adjustment and satisfaction, and less traditional sex-role behavior.[6]

Studies that examine the family backgrounds of voluntarily childless women offer different and at times conflicting interpretations of the effect of family background. Patterns of identification with parental figures are not consistent among voluntarily childless women. Sometimes both parents can be rejected as adult models. Sometimes mother is seen as a victim in some way and subsequently rejected as a female model. Other times father is seen as the more nurturant parent, which presumably makes him a more available identification for his daughter.[7] Low family warmth has been, however, the most frequent finding among families of women childless by choice. Permissive parental authority and parental encouragement of independence and achievement are also common findings among the families of voluntarily childless women.[8] In contrast to what might be expected, voluntarily childless women do not have mothers who are any more achievement oriented, nor are they more likely to be employed than the mothers of adult women who are also mothers.[9]

Veveers and Houseknecht, two women researchers who have done substantial research on childless women, have articulated two different categories of voluntary childlessness: the early deciders and the postponers.[10] Both define early deciders as those women who decide before the age of 30 that they are not going to have children. Although each researcher has identified a group of childless women as postponers, the characteristics of the definitions are quite different. Veveers describes the postponers as women who delay making a childbearing decision until it is too late. These women correspond more to the transitional women of the present study. Houseknecht's postponers, on the other hand, are women who show assertiveness and autonomy, and utilize support from a selected network of people to develop an alternative lifestyle which does not include motherhood. These women correspond more closely to the transformative women in this study.

Research on infertile or involuntarily childless women has not focused as much on how they may be different from women who are mothers, perhaps because they are seen as less deviant than women who *choose* not to have children. Rather, this research has focused on the depression, guilt, loss of female identity, and changed social interactions that are a part of the developmental crisis and mourning process that infertility can initiate.[11] In contrast to the voluntarily childless women, involuntarily childless women are more likely to have a feminine sex-role orientation; they more frequently endorse characteristics associated with a traditional female sex role. This sex-role orientation tends to make them more vulnerable to the loss of motherhood than are women who are less traditional, because one aspect of the traditional female role is being a mother. In a 1976 study, no significant differences between voluntarily and involuntarily childless women were found in such variables as socioeconomic status, religion, or marriage.[12] However, comparative studies between these two categories of childless women are limited.

About the Study

Selection of Women Interviewed

Women were selected from a pool of approximately 330 women who responded to two television news interviews (KGO, Channel 7,

June 23–24, 1988, with Anna Chavez) broadcast in Northern California and an article published in the San Jose *Mercury News* regarding this research study. Respondents were contacted by telephone and the focused in-depth interview procedure was explained. Consenting women were asked to complete a brief screening questionnaire that was mailed to them. These questionnaires were used to create the groupings.

One hundred women between the ages of 38 and 50 were selected and stratified into three groups: childless by choice, childless by delay, and childless by infertility or health problems. Group membership was defined in the following way. Group I (childless by choice) included those who, on the screening questionnaire, gave high ranks to items pertaining to making an active choice (whether early or late in life) to remain childless. High ranking of questionnaire items such as "never wanted children" or "childbearing conflicts with career goals or other values" warranted inclusion in Group I. Group II included those who gave high ranks to items relating to circumstances that created delay or made the decision more receptive than active. These questionnaire items include "postponed decision," "timing of relationships," "financial constraints," "mate did not want children," and "no mate." Group III included those who gave high ranks to items related to infertility ("genetically unable to conceive," "disease rendered pregnancy impossible," "other medical conditions made pregnancy dangerous," or "other—infertility of mate"). Employment characteristics, marital and racial characteristics, and pregnancy history of these three groups are summarized in Tables 1, 2, and 3.

TABLE 1. Employment Characteristics of Sample

	n	Professional	Nonprofessional	Unemployed	Student
Transformative (choice)	39	24	9	4	2
Transitional (delay)	32	16	11	2	3
Traditional (infertile)	31	14	12	3	2

TABLE 2. Marital and Racial Characteristics of Sample

	n	Married	Single	Cohabiting	Women of color	Cauca-sian	Other
Transformative (choice)	39	17	14	8	8	30	1
Transitional (delay)	32	7	22	3	8	23	1
Traditional (infertile)	31	21	7	3	9	22	—

Interviewing

At the time of the scheduled interview and prior to the initiation of the interview each subject completed the Bem Sex Role Inventory and signed a consent form. Because the Bem Sex Role Inventory has been shown to demonstrate that childless women have a nontraditional sex-role orientation, this study investigated possible differences among childless women in sex role orientation depending on the circumstances leading to their childlessness (choice, delay, infertility). The Bem data was submitted to a chi-square analysis.

The primary method of this research was the focused interview. This method emphasizes the discovery and illumination of concepts and theory through systematic analysis of data versus the logical deductive formulations of other approaches.[13] The focused in-depth interview allows flexibility as needed for unexpected data to emerge without premature closure, while concomitantly preventing aimless wandering during the interview. This

TABLE 3. Pregnancy History of Sample

	n	Abortions	Adoption	Miscarriage	Tubal pregnancy
Transformative (choice)	39	17	2	1	0
Transitional (delay)	32	19	1	1	0
Traditional (infertile)	31	9	1	1	1

TABLE 4. Bem Sex Role Inventory Results[a]

	n[b]	Feminine	Masculine	Androgynous	Undifferentiated
Transformative (choice)	35	2	**14**	4	**15**
Transitional (delay)	25	5	3	**13**	4
Traditional (infertile)	31	**10**	6	8	7

Note. Results in bold are significantly different from expected frequencies.
[a]Chi-square = 24.47, $p < .001$.
[b]11 subjects in the full sample did not complete the Bem Sex Role Inventory.

method provided structure for covering the same basic ground in all interviews and controlling the interview situation.[14]

Bem Sex Role Inventory Results

The Bem results for the entire sample of 100 women did not support prior research findings of a nontraditional sex-role orientation. Yet when the sample is stratified into the three groups of choice, delay, and infertility, significant findings did emerge (Table 4). The women who chose a child-free life more frequently exhibited a masculine or undifferentiated sex role. A masculine orientation reflects the focus needed for developing professional careers and in this situation may be correlated with a woman's ability to maintain a decision regarding a child-free life in the face of social expectations regarding motherhood. The occurrence of the number of women also selecting an undifferentiated orientation may suggest that for these women traditional gender-role characteristics are simply not prominent in their own self-perceptions. These women are actively challenging the assumption of deficiency and female inadequacy that childlessness implies.

The women who have become childless through a path of delay more frequently exhibited an androgynous orientation. Many of these women describe a long period of "coming of age," of exploring various activities developing themselves. For these women the theme of maternal ambivalence is present; their androgynous orientation may reflect the fact that the traditional masculine and feminine worlds are equally compelling to them.

The infertile women exhibited a feminine sex role more often than did either of the other two groups. Because infertility could be said to represent a biological rather than a psychological sampling, sex-role orientation appears to be less influential in their identity development than the fact of their infertility. These women, unlike the women childless by choice or delay, cannot say to themselves, "Well, I could have had a baby." As a result, in many of these women there can be a narcissistic blow to the self not wholly related to the woman's actual degree of maternal desire; this narcissistic wound must be repaired. The grief process also appears to be more profound for the women who are infertile and who identify with a feminine sex role.

Family of Origin Factors

The decision to remain childless, or the process of coming to terms with childlessness, is affected by family background, cultural influences, the nature of significant relationships, and the specific ways in which one redirects the creative energy previously reserved for the task of motherhood. A common negative myth is that all childless women must come from dysfunctional families.

All of the women interviewed here were members of the "baby boom" generation. They share a heritage of the myth of the nuclear family as it was portrayed in 1950s television programs like "Donna Reed" and "Ozzie and Harriet." Another aspect of their shared heritage may be the notion that, unless she suffers from infertility, only a woman from a "dysfunctional" family would remain childless. As noted earlier, research has indeed found certain negative characteristics, such as lower emotional warmth, in the families of voluntarily childless woman. Childless daughters have also been found to reject or, at best, only partially identify with mother as a female model.[15]

Most stereotypes contain within them a grain of truth, which is why they survive and are so difficult to dismiss. What is that grain here? Approximately one-quarter of the women childless by choice (transformative) and childless by delay (transitional), and slightly less than one-quarter of the women childless by infertility (traditional), described families in which a parent was significantly impaired by emotional problems or alcoholism. Dysfunctional parents were described as either overly or insufficiently invested in their children in such a way that parental responsibilities were not adequately fulfilled. In some families the interviewed daughter had stepped into a parental role, creating a situation where, in adulthood, the daughter felt she had not really been "seen" or nurtured in her family. Many of these daughters felt a need to repair an emotional deficit; they may have had reservations about motherhood stemming from fears of replicating their own damaging family experience. One 46-year-old transitional woman, the eldest of two daughters, said:

> *I got no parenting from my father. My father was a tyrant, a bully, loud and abusive. There was always a lot of guilt growing up because my father would use my mother as leverage with my sister and I. Whenever we did anything he didn't think was the right thing to do, he would hit my mother so he could pull us back in line. And whenever my mother did something he didn't particularly like he would kick the shit out of us. So he always kept an even balance, and he always kept us all in line and doing what he wanted us to do.*

This woman very much wanted to have children, but found herself repeatedly involved with unsuitable men—a pattern of relationship representing her unconscious efforts to work through unresolved issues with her dysfunctional father.

Marilyn, whose life is described in Chapter 4, was called on as the oldest of five siblings to fulfill many parental functions in her dysfunctional family:

> *By the time I was 10 or 12 it [mother's drinking] was severe and my father basically left around that time. My mother's drinking increased a lot when the marriage started to fall apart. And though he didn't totally abandon us, he was unpredictable. He had been the breadwinner, and now his financial situation was not good, and whether he would show up was always in the air, and whether he would have the money was up in the air.*

Family histories such as these do support the stereotype that dysfunctional families produce childless daughters. There is a paradox inherent within this stereotype; most daughters in dysfunctional families do become mothers. The paradox that dysfunctional families produce many more adults who are parents than childless adults is aptly expressed by a 46-year-old woman who decided in her 20s not to have a child. Three of her siblings now have children. Her decision grew out of an unexpected pregnancy that evoked disturbing dreams and many negative, painful emotional memories. With pain and humor she commented:

We [she and her siblings] talked about it and it wasn't so much a matter of why I didn't have children, but how could they have them after what we went through?

Most daughters in dysfunctional families grow up to become parents, often with the explicit intention of raising their children differently. They desire to repair and redo (through the parenting of their own children) the painful emotional residue of childhood. Support groups and writings about dysfunctional families popularized in recent years by the Adult Children of Alcoholics (ACOA) movement address the fact that becoming a parent in order to repair childhood trauma has only mixed success in resolving trauma. Sometimes the trauma is repeated with the former child taking on the role of her or his parent. Sometimes the dysfunctional pattern is repeated in some variation by choosing a mate who fulfills the role of the former parent. Other variations on the original dysfunctional family pattern can also occur. Having children with the expressed and conscious intention to do "better" than our own parents is no guarantee that this will, in fact, occur. Resolving childhood trauma or disappointments can be assisted by the inner psychological work that leads to awareness and understanding of the effects of these early experiences. The ACOA movement promotes this work.

Only one-quarter of the women interviewed described families of origin that could be termed "dysfunctional." These women exemplify the psychological strength and resiliency of women who forge a different path of adult development, rather than risk a repetition of dysfunctional family relationships.

Three-quarters of the interviewees described growing up in an "average, run of the mill" family—not perfect, but with a share of life's misfortunes, burdens, and less than ideal parenting. Most of the women grew up in intact families; only 17% had divorced parents. A 50-year-old transformative woman, the seventh of eight children in a Midwestern farming family, described her family in a way similar to many of the women with whom I spoke:

Daddy worked. He was the breadwinner. Period. And he
played with us. Momma did all the discipline. She didn't work
. . . well, she did work but she was at home with all the kids.
. . . She was Momma; she was there. She was there all the time.
We took Momma for granted.

Most of the women childless by choice (transformative) in my
study were able to identify a specific role within their families, and
40% of these women reported being the "parentified" child, or
caretaker in their families; this is a fairly common finding in
research on families of voluntarily childless women. There were
more eldest children in this group as well, another common finding
among voluntarily childless women.[16] Perhaps these women had
had enough of parenting for a lifetime! Another 20% of those
childless by choice identified a family role in which they were the
recipient of negative feelings from the parents. These women, who
were scapegoated by the family in childhood, at times perceived
their scapegoating as confirmation of their difference from the
mother; this negative difference did in part contribute to their
rejection of motherhood in later adult life. Thus the women who
choose not to become mothers seem often to be the *good* or *bad* child
in the family; we could say that they stood out in some noticeable
way.

However, 25% of the women childless by infertility (traditional) and by delay (transitional) also reported being the parental
child. Daughters, it seems, are much more likely to be placed in
parental roles. This is especially true if the daughter is the oldest
child and/or the only girl. But the meaning that this role has for the
daughter is not the same for all daughters! Though all the women
interviewed were childless, some found the parental role a fulfilling
one and looked forward to growing up to have children of their
own. Others used the nurturing skills they developed as caretakers
in other areas of their life. Still others simply left their caretaking in
the past and moved on to other things. Being a caretaker in her
family of origin does not indicate that a woman will remain
childless, although it may be a factor.

The majority of the women interviewed perceived their parents
as being neutral on the question of motherhood. This neutral, often
silent, position permitted the daughter to develop whatever

fantasies she may have had about her parents' experience. For some women the silence had a very positive emotional quality; a permission to live life as they saw fit. For others the silence left them with an uncertainty regarding the meaning and value of parenthood in their parents' lives and, by implication, their own.

When asked how they imagined their parents felt about being parents, most responded like the 45-year-old woman who said: "I think that they didn't really feel anything other than that is what you did. You grew up, you got married, and you had children. It was just what you did." Perhaps this comment reveals the changing cultural context between their generations. It was only in the daughters' generation that a real cultural space opened up for women (and men) to be able to consider seriously whether or not they wanted to become parents. These daughters had an opportunity to address the childbearing question that was not generally available to their mothers and fathers.

Because in most of these families there was at least one sibling who did grow up to become a parent, it would be reasonable to conclude that the values of these families are not very different from those of families whose adult children are parents. In fact, honesty and hard work were the most frequently mentioned values in all three groups—values that reflect the basic puritan values of many American families.

The women childless by choice (transformative) reported a slightly greater emphasis in their families on achievement than did women in the other two groups. This group included the greatest number of professional women. Previous studies of voluntarily childless women had shown independence to be a family value, and I had expected this group to value independence the most. However, it was the women childless by delay (transitional) who most frequently reported independence being valued in their families. An emphasis on interpersonal connection and a loving approach to others was also mentioned most frequently by these women. This pattern of conflicting values may have had an impact on these women's ambivalence and their feelings about the dual pursuit of family life and a life of their own, which they find hard to resolve.

Infertile (traditional) women also reported that their families valued independence. I have wondered if this may reflect an artifact of this particular study. Far fewer infertile women responded to the public interview requests. It may be that these particular women who were interviewed represent a special group of traditional women who have more completely resolved their infertile status. Valuing independence would no doubt help the traditional woman to shift her self-definition when she realizes that motherhood is not possible for her.

Another finding in all three groups was the noticeable absence of religion as a strong value. This has also been found in other studies of childless women.[17] We can speculate that families less identified with institutionalized religion may convey to their daughters less stereotypical attitudes about women and their roles.

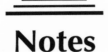

Notes

Chapter 1

1. It is impossible to know exactly what percentage of adult women beyond their childbearing years are childless; accurate statistics on these women are not recorded by the U. S. Census Bureau.
   Fertility of American women. U. S. Census Bureau, 1988.
2. Of the following recent books concerned with childless couples or the decision to remain childless, the work of Jane English takes childlessness out of a context of deviance and into one of transformation. Might this be a vision for the 21st century?
   Peck, E. (1971). *The baby trap*. New York: Bernard Geis.
   Veveers, J. (1972). *The violation of fertility mores: Voluntary childlessness as deviant behavior and societal reaction*. Toronto: Holt, Rinehart and Winston.
   Fabe, M., & Wikler, N. (1979). *Up against the clock*. New York: Random House.
   Faux, M. (1984). *Childlessness by choice*. New York: Anchor Press.
   Campbell, E. (1985). *The childless marriage*. London: Tavistock.
   English, J. (1989). *Childlessness transformed: Stories of alternative parenting*. Mount Shasta, CA: Earth Heart.
   Hunt, L. (1992). *Never to be a mother: A guide for women who didn't or couldn't have children*. San Francisco: Harper.
   Lang, S. (1991). *Women without children*. New York: Pharos Press.
3. The outpouring of public response to a single local television interview in which the author discussed her research regarding the lives of childless women illustrates the fact that this social absence is experienced by many women who are not mothers as emotionally painful and/or frustrating.
4. Tolnay, S., & Guest, A. (1982). Childlessness in a transitional population: The United States at the turn of the century. *Journal of Family History, Summer, 7*, 200–219.
   Fertility of American women. U. S. Census Bureau, 1988, 1990.

Westoff, C. (1986). Fertility in the United States. *Science, 2–4*, 549–554.

Boyd, R. (1989). Racial differences in childlessness: A centennial review. *Sociological Perspective, 32*, 183–199.

5. Rosie the Riveter was a World War II poster created and distributed by the U. S. Government to attract women into the workplace to support the war effort. Following the postwar decade of the 1950s, fertility again declined, hitting its lowest point in 1976.

Ryan, M. (1975). *Womanhood in America.* New York: New Viewpoints.

6. Gitlin, T. (1987). *The sixties: Years of hope, days of rage.* New York: Bantam.

7. For a discussion of the interface of postmodernist thought with psychoanalysis and feminism, see:

Flax, J. (1990). *Thinking fragments: Psychoanalysis, feminism and postmodernism in the contemporary west.* Berkeley, CA: University of California Press.

8. Gitlin, T. *The sixties: Years of hope, days of rage.* New York: Bantam.

9. Rubin, L. (1990). *The erotic wars: What ever happened to the sexual revolution?* New York: Farrar, Strauss & Giroux.

10. Dagg, P. (1991). The psychological sequelae of therapeutic abortion. *American Journal of Psychiatry, 148*, 578–585.

11. The abortion rights of women established in the 1973 Supreme Court decision (Roe vs. Wade) undermined by the 1989 decision granting states greater latitude in limiting abortions and the 1991 decision prohibiting federally funded clinics from dispensing information on abortion are being reversed by the Clinton administration. This direction supports the United Nations Worldwatch Institute's findings that "restrictions on pregnancy terminations do not curb abortion rates; they only cause more deaths" for women. See:

Sinai, R. (1990, July 15). *Oakland Tribune.*

12. It is impossible to know exactly what percentage of adult women beyond their childbearing years are childless; accurate statistics on these women are not recorded by the U. S. Census Bureau.

Fertility of American women. U. S. Census Bureau, 1988.

13. Chanter, T. (1990). Female temporality and the future of feminism. In J. Fletcher & A. Benjamin (Eds.), *Abjection, melancholia, and love: The work of Julia Kristeva* (pp. 63–80). New York: Routledge.

14. Tolnay, S., & Guest, A. (1982). Childlessness in a transitional population: The United States at the turn of the century. *Journal of Family History, Summer, 7*, 200–219.

15. Of the women interviewed for this study, 74% of the "traditional" women, 64% of the "transitional" women, and 46% of the "transformative" women mentioned relationships as a significant shaping influence.

16. For a readable discussion of female–male differences, see:
    Rubin, L. (1985). *Just friends* New York: Harper & Row.
17. In the three categories, the following percentages of women said that friendships were very significant in their lives: "traditional" women, 59%; "transitional" women, 65%; "transformative" women, 59%.
18. For a discussion of the interface of declining birthrate and women entering the workforce as one among many variables affecting contemporary motherhood, see:
    Gerson, K. (1985). *Hard choices: How women decide about work, career, and motherhood.* Berkeley, CA: University of California Press.
19. These are the women whom Veveers describes as "postponers," women who delay making a decision regarding childbearing until it is too late. See:
    Veveers, J. E. (1973). Voluntary childlessness: A neglected area of family study. *Family Coordinator, 22,* 199–205.
20. Houseknecht uses the term "postponers" to describe this group of childless women; women who show assertiveness, autonomy, and who utilize support from a selected network of people to uphold an alternative lifestyle which does not include motherhood. See:
    Houseknecht, S. K. (1979). Reference group support for voluntary childless wives. *Social Biology, 23,* 198–109.

Chapter 2

1. The biographical material in this and the following chapters is drawn from in-depth interviews conducted in 1988 with 100 childless women. Follow-up information was obtained 3 years later from the interviewees.
2. Developed by Sandra Bem, the Bem Sex Role Inventory (BSRI) is a list of adjectives, some of which are characteristic of a feminine sex role, some of the male sex role, and others neutral. Individuals rate themselves according to the degree to which the adjective describes them (almost never true to almost always true). The instrument was extensively used in feminist research of the 1970s, correlating sex role orientation with a number of psychological variables.
    Bem, S. (1974). The measurement of psychological androgyny. *Journal of Consulting and Clinical Psychology, 42,* 155–162.

Responses to the BSRI were grouped into one of four personality styles: masculine, feminine, androgynous, or undifferentiated. The concept of androgyny, a personality style seen as exhibiting characteristics of both sexes, and combining the best of male and female roles, was a popular one at the time.

Singer, J. (1976) *Androgyny: Toward a new psychology of sexuality*. New York: Anchor Press.

For Bem's later thoughts on the concept of androgyny in gender schema theory and its implications for child development, see:
Bem, S. (1983). Raising gender-aschematic children in a gender schematic society. *Signs: Journal of Women in Culture and Society, 8,* 598–616.

3. *Infertility: Medical and social choices.* (1988). Washington, DC: Office of Technology Assessment.
4. Burch, B. (1989). Mourning and failure to mourn: An object-relations view. *Contemporary Psychoanalysis, 25,* 608–623.

For resources, see:
Becker, G. (1990). *Healing the infertile family.* New York: Bantam.
Hunt, L. (1992). *Never to be a mother.* San Francisco: Harper & Row.
5. Freud, S. (1917). Mourning and melancholia. *Standard Edition, 14,* 243–260. London: Hogarth Press.

Chapter 3

1. "Transitional" women scored significantly higher in the "androgynous" category on the Bem Sex Role Inventory than did either the "traditional" or "transformative" women.
2. If the woman is heterosexual, she can't quite decide if she wants a traditional mate and provider or a more liberated male as her partner. If she is homosexual, she can't quite decide what circumstances she needs to support her bearing and raising a child.
3. Markus, H., & Nurius, P. (1986). Possible selves. *American Psychologist, 41,* 954–969.
4. For a more complete understanding of this idea, see:
Raglund-Sullivan, E. (1987). *Jacques Lacan and the philosophy of psychoanalysis.* Chicago: Univeristy of Illinois Press.
5. In psychoanalytic terms the process of perceiving in others denied aspects of one's self is known as projection. For a development of Melanie Klein's fertile concept of the process of projective identification in relationships and identity development, see:
Ogden, T. (1981). *Projective identification.* New York: Aronson.

For a discussion of how these processes operate in couples, see:
Bader, E., & Pearson, P. (1988). *In quest of the mythical mate: Diagnosing the treating of the developmental stages of couplehood.* New York: Brunner/Mazel.

Obviously women who are mothers must also come to grips with their projections upon men, but it is perhaps easier to avoid doing so because stereotypical parental roles tend to support mutual projection.

6. For a Jungian perspective on a woman's process of integrating her own competencies through becoming related to her animus, see:

   Young-Eisendrath, P., & Wiedemann, F. L. (1987). *Female authority: Empowering women through psychotherapy.* New York: Guilford Press.

Chapter 4

1. For the correlation of "masculine" traits and psychological well-being and a general discussion of the controversy over the 1970s idealization of androgyny, see:

   Taylor, M. C., & Hall, J. A., (1982). Psychological androgyny: Theories, methods, and conclusions. *Psychological Bulletin, 92,* 347–366.

2. Ehrensaft, D. (1987). *Parenting together: Men and women sharing the care of their children.* New York: Free Press.

3. Women who make an early (teens or 20s) decision to remain child-free are more frequently reacting to a dysfunctional family background than women who decide later. A dysfunctional family is one in which the emotional problems of the parent(s) significantly interfere with the capacity to fulfill parental responsibilities.

4. It is a common consequence of divorce that a divorced woman's standard of living goes down substantially whereas that of the ex-husband goes up. For a critical perspective on the family, divorce, children, and feminism, see:

   Hewlett, S. A. (1987). *A lesser life.* New York: Warner.

5. Bram, S. (1984). Voluntarily childless women: Traditional or nontraditional? *Sex Roles, 10,* 195–206.

   Bram, S. (1986). Childlessness revisited: A longitudinal study of voluntarily childless couples, delayed parents, and parents. *Lifestyles: A Journal of Changing Patterns, 3,* 46–65.

   Houseknecht, S. K. (1978). A social psychological model of voluntary childlessness. *Alternative Lifestyles, I,* 379–402.

Thirty-eight percent of the transformative women were or had been significantly involved with friends' children; 45% of the traditional women and 32% of the transitional women reported such involvement.

Chapter 5

1. Freud, S. (1931). Female sexuality. *Standard Edition, 21,* 223–226. London: Hogarth Press.

2. Freud, S. (1925). Some psychical consequences of the anatomical distinction between the sexes. *Standard Edition, 19*, 248–260. London: Hogarth Press.
3. Deutsch, H. (1969). The significance of masochism in the mental life of women. In R. Fleiss (Ed.), *The psychoanalytic reader* (pp. 195–207). New York: International Universities Press. (Original work published 1930.)
4. Freud, S. (1924). The economic problem of masochism. *Standard Edition, 19*, 159–172. London: Hogarth Press.
5. Young-Bruehl, E. (1990). *Freud on women: A reader.* New York: Norton.
6. Horney, K. (1933). *The problem of feminine masochism.* New York: Norton.
   Klein, M. (1928). Early stages of the oedipus complex. *International Journal of Psycho-Analysis, 9*, 167–180.
7. Horney, K. (1924). On the genesis of the castration complex in women. *International Journal of Psycho-Analysis, 5*, 50–65.
   Jones, E. (1961). Early development of female sexuality (original publication date 1927) and Early female sexuality (original publication date 1935). In *Papers on psychoanalysis.* (pp. 438–451; 485–495). Boston: Beacon Press.
8. Horney, K. (1926). The flight from womanhood: The masculinity complex in women as viewed by men and women. *International Journal of Psycho-Analysis, 7*, 324–339.
9. For an excellent elaboration of Horney's work, see:
   Weskott, M. (1986). *The feminist legacy of Karen Horney.* New Haven, CT: Yale University Press.
10. Golden, C. (in press). *A new psychology of women.* New York: Guilford Press.
11. Kleeman, J. (1976). Freud's views on early female sexuality in the light of direct child observation. *Journal of the American Psychoanalytic Association, 24*, 3–27.
    Bernstein, D. (1990). Female genital anxieties, conflicts, and typical modes. *International Journal of Psycho-Analysis, 71*, 151–165.
12. Masters, W. H., & Johnson, V. E. (1966). *Human sexual response.* Boston: Little Brown.
13. Sherfey, M. (1966). The evolution and nature of female sexuality in relation to psychoanalytic theory. *Journal of the American Psychoanalytic Association, 14*, 28–128.
    Fliegel, Z. (1986). Women's development in analytic theory: Six decades of controversy. In J. Alpert (Ed.), *Psychoanalysis and women: Contemporary reappraisals* (pp. 3–33). Hillsdale, NJ: Analytic Press.
    Dujoven, B. (1991). Contemporary revisions of classical psychoanalytic theory of early female development. *Psychotherapy, 28*, 317–326.

14. Parens, H., Polock, L., Stern, J., & Kramer, S. (1977). On the girl's entry into the oedipus complex. In H. P. Blum (Ed.), *Female psychology: Contemporary psychoanalytic views* (pp. 79–107). New York: International Universities Press.
15. Money, J., & Ehrhardt, A. (1982). *Man and woman: Boy and girl.* Baltimore, MD: John Hopkins University Press.
16. See Robert Stoller's work on core gender identity, including:
    Stoller, R. (1965). The sense of maleness. *Psychoanalytic Quarterly, 34,* 207–218.
    Stoller, R. (1968). The sense of femaleness. *Psychoanalytic Quarterly, 37,* 42–55.
    Stoller, R. (1976). Primary femininity. *Journal of the American Psychoanalytic Association, 24,* 59–78.
    Stoller, R. (1980). Femininity. In M. Kirkpatrick (Ed.), *Women's sexual development.* New York: Plenum Press.
17. Stern, D. (1985). *The interpersonal world of the infant: A view from psychoanalysis and development psychology.* New York: Basic.
18. Fast, I. (1984). *Gender identity.* Hillsdale, NJ: Analytic Press.
19. Chodorow, N. (1978). *The reproduction of mothering.* Berkeley, CA: University of California Press.
    Chodorow, N. (1989). *Feminism and psychoanalytic theory.* New Haven, CT: Yale University Press.
20. Miller, J. B. (1976). *Toward a new psychology of women.* Boston: Beacon Press.
    Jordan, J., Kaplan, A., Miller, J., Stiver, I., & Surrey, J. (1991). *Women's growth in connection: Writings from the Stone Center.* New York: Guilford Press.

    In *Feminism and Psychoanalytic Theory* (see note 19, this chapter) Nancy Chodorow refers to the Stone Center writers as the "interpersonal group," to differentiate them from object-relational theorists. This term can be confusing, because "interpersonalist" has a particular meaning in psychoanalytic theory, specifically the views of Harry Stack Sullivan.
21. The object-relational paradigm of W. R. D. Fairbairn offers a model of development beginning with the dependency of infancy to the quasi-independence of childhood and adolescence to the mutual interdependency of adulthood. Clearly developmental theory has focused too much on the individuation process and neglected the concept of mutual interdependence. This neglected aspect has been the focus of the Stone Center, but we must ask whether it is of benefit for all women (or men) to frame mutuality and interdependency specifically in female terms. Can the apparent inability of many boys to move from quasi-independence to mutual dependence be thought of as a result of

their need to relinquish early maternal identification in order to develop a different gender identity from mother? Perhaps mutual interdependency is simply more obvious in the development of females because it is more readily achieved due to the girl's unabandoned maternal identification.

22. Gilligan, C. (1982). *In a different voice*. Cambridge, MA: Harvard University Press.
23. Belenky, M., Clinchy, B., Goldberger, N., & Tarule, J. (1986). *Women's ways of knowing: The development of self, voice, and mind*. New York: Basic.
24. Gilligan, C. (1991, January, 9). Survey finds girls have poor self image. *San Francisco Chronicle*. p. 8.

This research shows significant racial differences, with black girls retaining more self-esteem than white or Hispanic girls. This may be because black girls are often surrounded by strong women they admire.
25. Hancock, E. (1989). *The girl within*. New York: Dutton.
26. Lacan, J. (1977) *Ecrits*. New York: Norton.
Lacan, J. (1978) *Four fundamental concepts of psychoanalysis*. New York: Norton.
Lacan, J. (1985) *Feminine sexuality*. New York: Norton
27. Raglund-Sullivan, E. (1987). *Jacques Lacan and the philosophy of psychoanalysis*. Chicago: University of Illinois Press.
Felman, S. (1987). *Jacques Lacan and the adventure of insight*. Cambridge, MA: Harvard University Press.
Tamsin, L. (1990). *Gender identity and the production of meaning: Feminist theory and politics*. Boulder, CO: Westview Press.
28. Irigaray, L. (1985). *This sex which is not one*. Ithaca, NY: Cornell University Press.
Irigaray, L. (1985). *Speculum of the other woman*. Ithaca, NY: Cornell University Press.
Irigaray, L. (1991). *The marine lover of Frederich Nietsche*. New York: Columbia University Press.
Whiteford, M. (1991). *Luce Irigaray: Philosophy in the feminine*. London: Routledge.
30. Moi, T. (Ed.). (1986). *The Kristeva reader*. New York: Columbia University Press.
Fletcher, J., & Benjamin, A., (Eds.). (1990). *Abjection, melancholia, and love: The work of Julia Kristeva*. London: Routledge.
31. Gallop, J. (1988). *Thinking through the body*. New York: Columbia University Press.
Gallop, J. (1982). *The daughter's seduction: Feminism and psychoanalysis*. Ithaca, NY: Cornell University Press.

32. Benjamin, J. (1988). *The bonds of love: Psychoanalysis, feminism and the problem of domination*. New York: Pantheon.
33. Chasseguet-Smirgel, J. (1976). Freud and female sexuality: The consideration of some blind spots in the exploration of the 'dark continent.' *International Journal of Psycho-Analysis, 57*, 275–286.

Chapter 6

1. Fliegel, Z. (1986). Women's development in analytic theory: Six decades of controversy. In J. Alpert (Ed.), *Women and psychoanalysis: Contemporary perspectives* (pp. 3–33). Hillsdale, NJ: Analytic Press.
2. Chodorow suggests that the usual separation–individuation process of the child, male or female, can distort the child's emerging identity when the mother's access to other validating social roles is significantly restricted by a patriarchal society; as a result of this restriction the mother can become overly and instrusively invested in her children.
3. Winnicott, D. W. (1971). *Playing and reality*. London: Tavistock.

Freud also originally made bisexuality a cornerstone of psychoanalytic theory, and then moved away from this position, putting the female baby in the position of being a "little man" before she develops her female identification. The feminist–analyst Julia Kristeva argues that grounding identity in bisexuality provides for the possibility of representation or signification in language of the full range of female and male experience.
Kristeva, J. (1981). Oscillation between power and denial. In E. Marks & I. de Courtivron (Eds.), *New French feminisms* (165–168). New York: Schoken.
4. The child's sexuality is split, with one aspect of sexuality becoming more or less repressed, resulting in either a heterosexual or homosexual orientation.
5. Stern, D. (1985). *The interpersonal world of the infant*. New York: Basic.
6. For further development of mother's subjectivity, see:
Benjamin, J. (1988). *The bonds of love*: Psychoanalysis, feminism, and the problem of domination. New York: Pantheon.
7. For a description of this process, see the chapters, "On the use of the object" and "Relating through identifications" in:
Winnicott, D. W. (1971). *Playing and reality*. London: Tavistock.
8. Benjamin, J. (1988). *The bonds of love*: Psychoanalysis, feminism, and the problem of domination. New York: Pantheon.
9. I am indebted to Joyce McDougall for this metaphor:
McDougall, J. (1985). *Theatres of the mind*. New York: Basic.

10. For a thoughtful presentation of the difficulties for the female child's identity development when she turns to father, see:

Benjamin, J. (1988). *The bonds of love: Psychoanalysis, feminism, and the problem of domination*.New York: Pantheon.

11. Lacan, J. (1977). *Ecrits*. New York: Norton.

Lacan, J. (1978). *The four fundamental concepts of psychoanalysis*. New York: Norton.

12. In classical psychoanalytic theory what this means, then, is that even when the infancy relationship with the mother is a satisfying one, when the female child enters the oedipal period, she will find that femaleness is devalued and maleness overvalued seemingly because father (male) has the penis and mother (female) does not—and, of course, neither does she. Given the positive cultural meanings that have become confused with the penis, the unfortunate outcome of this entire scenario is that a female child all too soon learns she is able to assume social authority only through her attachment to a man, who has the penis she lacks, and ultimately by having his child as some sort of phallic substitute. For a more complete discussion of the privileging of the visual sense in psychoanalysis and the problem of this phallus, see:

Gallop, J. (1982). *The daughter's seduction: Feminism and psychoanalysis*. Ithaca, NY: Cornell University Press.

13. For work concerning how women must write themselves into history if they are to be a part of it, see:

Wright, E. (1989). *Between feminism and psychoanalysis*. New York: Routledge.

For a provocative essay referring to both women's writing and inherent bisexuality, see:

Cixous, H. (1980). The laugh of the Medusa. E. Marks & I. de Courtivron, (Eds.), *New French feminisms* (pp. 245–265). New York: Schocken.

14. Winnicott does not see the father functioning exactly as does Lacan, but he does see the father functioning as a representative of the "whole" or individuated self toward which the child strives.

Winnicott, D. W. (1989). The use of an object in the context of Moses and monotheism. *Psychoanalytic explorations*. Cambridge, MA: Harvard University Press).

15. Winnicott, D. W., Ego distortion in terms of the true and false self (Maturational processes in the facilitating environment) and Mirror-role of mother and family in child development (Playing and reality).

16. Winnicott, D. W. (1971). On transitional objects and transitional phenomenon. *Playing and reality*.

See also Tom Ogden's elaboration of Winnicott's work in:

Ogden, T. (1986). *The matrix of the mind: Object-Relations and the psychoanalytic dialogue*. New York: Aronson.

17. Erickson, E. (1968). *Identity: Youth and crisis*. New York: Norton.
18. See such feminists as:

Chodorow, N. (1989). *Feminism and psychoanalytic theory*. New Haven, CT: Yale University Press.

Flax, J. (1990). *Thinking fragments: Psychoanalysis, feminism, and postmodernism in the contemporary West*. Berkeley, CA: University of California Press.

Harris, A. (1991). Gender as contradiction. *Psychoanalytic Dialogues, 1*, 197–224.

19. Irigaray suggests that females are positioned differently than men to the death drive because of their biological capacity to bear a life, sustain a life, or end a life. Because of this uniquely female capacity, whether it is exercised or not, women are in a different psychic relationship to death than are men who do not have this same biological capacity. As such female aggression cannot fully be managed or mediated through the institutions of western religion, which assist men in mediating their own aggression, because these have masculine godheads. See Margaret Whitford's discussion of Irigaray's ideas in:

Whitford, M. (1991). *Luce Irigaray: Philosophy in the feminine*. London: Routledge.

The multiplicity of women's sexuality is presented in:

Irigaray, L. (1985). *This sex which is not one*. Ithaca, NY: Cornell University Press.

The rise in popularity of the "Goddess" worship could be seen as an effort by women at this time to embrace a godhead that includes both the positive and negative aspects of aggression within the divine so this kind of mediation of aggression becomes possible. See:

Engelsman, J. (1987). *The feminine dimension of the divine*. Wilmette, IL: Chronicle.

20. Lerner, H. (1988). *Women in therapy*. Northvale, NJ: Aronson.
21. Chodorow, N. (1989). *Feminism and psychoanalytic theory*. New Haven, CT: Yale University Press.

Benjamin, J. (1988). *Bonds of Love: Psychoanalysis, feminism and thd problem of domination*. New York: Pantheon.

Chapter 7

1. For an accessible presentation of these ideas, see:

Raglund-Sullivan, E. R. (1987). *Jacques Lacan and the philosophy of psychoanalysis*. Chicago: University of Illinois Press.

Jessica Benjamin's *Bonds of love* uses the idea of the "third term" in female development.

2. Scott, J. (1990). Deconstructing equality versus difference: The uses of poststructuralist theory for feminism. In M. Hirsch & E. Keller, (Eds.), *Conflicts in feminism* (pp. 134–148). New York: Routledge.

3. Harris, A. (1991). Gender as contradiction. *Psychoanalytic Dialogues, 1,* 197–224.

4. American Psychiatric Association. (1987). *Diagnostic and statistical manual of mental disorders* (3rd ed., rev.). Washington, DC: Author.

5. Freud, S. (1920). Beyond the pleasure principle. *Standard Edition, 18,* 7–17. London: Hogarth Press.

6. For a discussion of the complexity of issues around surrogacy and the female body, see:
Eisenstein, Z. (1988). *The female body and the law*. Berkeley, CA: University of California Press.

7. For an excellent discussion of procreative technologies and the issues they raise, see:
Rothman, B. (1989). *Re-inventing motherhood*. New York: Norton.

8. Freud, S. (1931). Female sexuality. *Standard Edition, 21,* 223–226. London: Hogarth Press.

As noted in Chapter 5, Freud commented that women are made and not born, because females have to go through a process of shifting their primary love object from a female (mother) to a male (father). The research of John Money at Johns Hopkins, however, provides a more comprehensive view of gender as a social construction. Children who are born with chromosomal or genital malformations can be assigned a gender identity in early infancy that is not necessarily biologically congruent. But if this child is treated consistently as of either male or female gender by parents (or other caretakers), the child will assume that gender identity as part of their developing identity. See:
Money, J., & Ehrhardt, A. (1973). *Man and woman, boy and girl: Differentiation and dimorphism of gender identity from conception to maturity*. Baltimore, MD: Johns Hopkins University Press.

9. Faludi, S. (1991). *Backlash: The undeclared war against American women*. New York: Crown.

10. Winnicott, D. W. (1971). *Playing and reality*. New York: Basic.

See in particular "The use of the object" and "Relating through identifications."

11. Irigaray, L. (1985). *The sex which is not one*. Ithaca, NY: Cornell University Press.

12. For provocative discussions of this and related issues, see:
    Silverman, K. (1988). *Acoustic mirror*. Blomington, IN: Indiana University Press.
    Butler, J. (1990). *Gender trouble: Feminism and subversion of identity*. New York: Routledge.
13. As an example of this new focus, see:
    Jordan, J., Kaplan, A., & Surrey, J. (1990). *Empathy revisited* (Work in Progress, No. 40). Wellesley, MA: Stone Center.
    Nodding, N. (1990). Ethics from the standpoint of women. In D. Rhode (Ed.), *Theoretical perspectives on sexual difference* (pp. 160–173). New Haven, CT: Yale University Press.
14. Acceptance of the fluidity that characterizes the relationships of childless couples is illustrated in a phrase from Murray Stein: "Journeying is the best condition for loving."
    Stein, M. (1983). *In midlife: A Jungian perspective* Dallas, TX: Spring.

    A liminal space is implied in:
    Dimen, M. (1991). Deconstructing difference: Gender, splitting, and transitional space. *Psychoanalytic dialogues, 1*, 335–352.
15. For an excellent exploration of this theme, see:
    Flax, J. (1990). *Thinking fragments: Psychoanalysis, feminism, postmodernism in the contemporary West*. Berkeley, CA: University of California Press.
16. Winnicott, D. W. (1971). On transitional objects and transitional phenomenon. *Playing and reality*. New York: Basic.
17. For a look at midlife identity issues among women who are mothers, see:
    Rubin, L (1979). *Women of a certain age: The midlife search for self*. New York: Harper & Row.
18. For a discussion of the "misrecognition" idea—thinking we are what we have become identified with in others, see:
    Lacan, J. (1977). *Ecrits*. New York: Norton.
    Stein, M. (1983). *In midlife: A Jungian perspective*. Dallas, TX: Spring.
19. This concept is implied in object-relations theorist Tom Ogden's work, especially in his article regarding the dialectic of conscious–unconscious: Ogden, T. (in press). The dialectically constituted–decentered subject of psychoanalysis: Part I. The Freudian subjects; Part II. The contributions of Klein and Winnicott. *International Journal of Psycho-Analysis*.
20. See Chapter 6, on Julia Kristeva, and also:
    Elliott, P. (1991). *From mastery to analysis: Theories of gender in psychoanalysis*. Ithaca, NY: Cornell University Press.
    Fletcher, J., & Benjamin, A. (Eds.). (1990). *Abjection, melancholia, and love: The work of Julia Kristeva*. London: Routledge.

21. The Möbius strip is one of the topographical symbols Lacan uses in developing ideas. See:

Lacan, J. (1978). *The four fundamental concepts of psychoanalysis*. New York: Norton.

22. Fliegel, Z. (1986). Women's development in analytic theory: Six decades of controversy. In J. Alpert (Ed.), *Woman and psychoanalysis: Contemporary reappraisals* (pp. 3–33). Hillsdale, NJ: Analytic Press.

In classical theory, bearing a child (especially a male child) is a woman's compensation for not having the valued penis. In contrast, Janine Chassequet-Smirgel develops the feminist analytic view in which maternity in female identity is valued on its own terms, rather than as a compensation.

Chassequet-Smirgel, J. (1986). Freud and female sexuality: The consideration of some blind spots in the exploration of the "dark continent." In *Sexuality and mind*. New York: New York University Press.

Both views leave out women who aren't mothers.

23. Freud, S. (1925). Some psychical consequences of the anatomical distinction between the sexes. *Standard Edition, 19*, 248–260. London: Hogarth Press.

Chapter 8

1. Bollas, C. (1987). *The shadow of the object: Psychoanalysis of the unthought known*. New York: Columbia University Press.

In a presentation regarding women's reproductive life cycle, psychologist Sue Elkind has utilized Bollas' concept of the "unthought known" to characterize the female experience of reproductive life transitions.

2. "Lilith is the consciousness of absolute equality of male and female in the sight of God. The equality is reinforced by potential androgyny within each."

Begg, E. (1984). *Myth and today's consciousness*. London: Coventure.

The story of Lilith is drawn from this and the following sources:

Collona, M. T. (1980). Lilith or the black moon. *Journal of Analytical Psychology, 25*, 325–350.

Hurwitz, S. (1992). *Lilith: The first Eve*. Einsiedeln, Switzerland: Daimon Press.

Vogelsang, E. W. (1985). The confrontation between Lilith and Adam: The fifth round. *Journal of Analytical Psychology, 30*, 149–163.

3. One might view the intensity with which some women pursue

motherhood in the face of infertility, leading to the rise of surrogate births and in vitro fertilization as due in part to the inability of these women to perceive themselves as "real women" other than in a maternal identification. Although this limited self-definition is supported and reinforced by technological advances, these same advances and their implications for the meaning of motherhood also (paradoxically) contribute to its deconstruction.

4. While the 1992 Republican presidential campaign theme of family values appeared to be a move toward further gender entrenchment, the election of Democrat Bill Clinton (with Hillary) harbingers a period of progressive gender role thinking.

Appendix

1. Allison, J. R. (1979). Roles and role conflict of women in infertile couples. *Psychology of Women Quarterly, 4*, 97.
2. Sharon Houseknecht summarizes and reviews many of the studies on women's childlessness:
   Houseknecht, S. (1987). Voluntary childnessness. In M. B. Sussman & S. K. Steinmetz (Eds.), *Handbook of marriage and family* (pp. 369–395). New York: Plenum Press.

   Whereas childlessness in women may be beginning to be seen from perspectives other than deviance or pathology, this may not be so reassuring when taken together with the reality that women (childless or not) are over-represented as clients seeking help in mental health clinics, as noted in:
   Chesler, P. (1972). *Women and madness.* New York: Avon.
3. Baber, K. M. (1984). Delayed childbearing: The psychosocial aspects of the decision-making process. *Dissertation Abstracts International, 44* (ADD84-24411). University of Connecticut.
   Bram, S. (1984). Voluntarily childless woman: Traditional or nontraditional? *Sex Roles, 10*, 195–206.
   Cohen, L. S. (1985). The intention to remain childless: Separation response, sex-role identity and family background. *Dissertation Abstracts International, 45* (ADD84-24411) Michigan State University.
   Greenglass, E. R., & Borovilos. T. (1985) Psychological correlates of fertility plans in unmarried women. *Canadian Journal of Behavioral Sciences Review, 17*, 130–139.
4. Baum, F., & Cope, D. R. (1980). Some characteristics of intentionally childless wives in Britain. *Journal of Biosocial Science, 12*, 287–299.
   Bram, S. (1986). Childlessness revisited: A longitudinal study of

voluntarily childless couples, delayed parents, and parents. *Lifestyles: A Journal of Changing Patterns, 3,* 46–65.

Burman, B., & deAnela, D. (1986). Parenthood or nonparenthood: A comparison of intentional families. *Lifestyles: A Journal of Changing Patterns, 6,* 69–79.

Magarick, R. H. & Brown, R. A. (1981). Social and emotional aspects of voluntary childlessness in vasectomized childless men. *Journal of Biosocial Science, 13,* 34–42.

Silka, L., & Kiesler, S. (1977). Couples who choose to remain childless. *Family Planning Perspectives, 9,* 16–25.

5. For a summary and review of studies on women's childlessness, see:

Houseknecht, S. (1987). Voluntary childlessnessness. In M. B. Sussman & S. K. Steinmetz (Eds.), *Handbook of marriage and family* (pp. 369–395). New York: Plenum Press.

6. Feldman, H. (1981). A comparison of intentional parents and intentionally childless couples. *Journal of Marriage and the Family, 43,* 593–600.

Houseknecht, S. K. (1977). Reference group support for voluntary childlessness: Evidence for conformity. *Journal of Marriage and the Family, 39,* 285–292.

See also Lisowski (1981), Note 7 (Appendix), and Wilk (1986), Note 15 (Appendix).

7. Lisowski, S. J. (1981). A study of the father–daughter relationship in childhood: Its effects upon women's decisions involving motherhood and career. *Dissertation Abstracts International, 45,* (April, 10–B). University of Wisconsin.

Ward, L. M. (1983). Innovative female identity: Experiential antecedents of the capacity for nontraditional childbearing choices. *Dissertation Abstracts International, 44* (ADD83-19947). Boston University School of Education.

8. Cohen, L. S. (1985). The intention to remain childless: Separation response, sex-role identity and family background. *Dissertation Abstracts International, 45* (ADD84-24411). Michigan State University.

9. Veveers, J. E. (1971). The child-free alternative: Rejection of the motherhood mystique. In M. Stephenson (Ed.), *Women in Canada.* Toronto: New Press.

10. Houseknecht, S. K. (1979). Reference group support for voluntarily childless wives. *Social Biology, 23,* 98–109.

Veevers, J. E. (1973). Voluntary childlessness: A neglected area of family study. *Family Coordinator, 22,* 199–205.

11. Allison, J. R. (1979). Roles and role conflict of women in infertile couples. *Psychology of Women Quarterly, 4,* 97.

Kraft, A. D., Palombo, J., Mitchell, D., Dean, C., Meyers, S., & Schmidt, A. (1980). The psychological dimensions of infertility. *American Journal of Orthopsychiatry, 50,* 618–628.

McEwan, K. L., Costello, C. G., & Taylor, P. J. (1987). Adjustment to infertility. *Journal of Abnormal Psychology, 96,* 108–116.

Slade, P. (1981). Sexual attitudes and social role orientations in infertile women. *Journal of Psychosomatic Research, 46,* 183–186.

12. Poston, D. G. (1976). Characteristics of voluntarily and involuntarily childless wives. *Social Biology, 23,* 198–209.

13. Glaser, B. G., & Strauss, H. (1967). *The discovery of grounded theory: Strategies for qualitative research.* Chicago: Aldine.

14. Focused in-depth interview has been used extensively by Lilian Rubin in her work.

   Rubin, L. B. (1985). *Just friends: The role of friendship in our lives.* New York: Harper and Row.

   Rubin, L. B. (1983). *Intimate strangers: Men and women together.* New York: Harper and Row.

   Rubin, L. B. (1979). *Women of a certain age: The midlife search for self.* New York: Harper and Row.

   Rubin, L. B. (1976). *Worlds of pain: Life in the working-class family.* New York: Basic.

15. Wilk, C. (1986). *Career women and childbearing: A psychological analysis of the decision process.* New York: Van Nostrand Reinhold.

16. Nason, E. M., & Paloma, M. M. (1976). *Voluntarily childless couples.* Beverly Hills, CA: Sage.

17. Xoustauzis, S. O., & Henley, J. R. (1971). Correlates of voluntary childlessness in a select population. *Social Biology, 18,* 277–284.

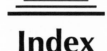

Index